Issues in Transplant Surgery

Editor

JUAN M. PALMA-VARGAS

SURGICAL CLINICS OF NORTH AMERICA

www.surgical.theclinics.com

Consulting Editor
RONALD F. MARTIN

February 2019 • Volume 99 • Number 1

ELSEVIER

1600 John F. Kennedy Boulevard • Suite 1800 • Philadelphia, Pennsylvania, 19103-2899

http://www.surgical.theclinics.com

SURGICAL CLINICS OF NORTH AMERICA Volume 99, Number 1
February 2019 ISSN 0039–6109, ISBN-13: 978-0-323-65519-4

Editor: John Vassallo, j.vassallo@elsevier.com
Developmental Editor: Meredith Madeira

Surgical Clinics of North America (ISSN 0039–6109) is published bimonthly by Elsevier Inc., 360 Park Avenue South, New York, NY 10010-1710. Months of publication are February, April, June, August, October, and December. Business and Editorial Offices: 1600 John F. Kennedy Blvd., Suite 1800, Philadelphia, PA 19103-2899. Periodicals postage paid at New York, NY and additional mailing offices. Subscription prices are $417.00 per year for US individuals, $845.00 per year for US institutions, $100.00 per year for US students and residents, $507.00 per year for Canadian individuals, $1071.00 per year for Canadian institutions, $536.00 for international individuals, $1071.00 per year for international institutions and $250.00 per year for Canadian and foreign students/residents. To receive student/resident rate, orders must be accompanied by name of affiliated institution, date of term, and the *signature* of program/residency coordinator on institution letterhead. Orders will be billed at individual rate until proof of status is received. Foreign air speed delivery is included in all *Clinics* subscription prices. All prices are subject to change without notice. POSTMASTER: Send address changes to *Surgical Clinics*, Elsevier Health Sciences Division, Subscription Customer Service, 3251 Riverport Lane, Maryland Heights, MO 63043. **Customer Service (orders, claims, online, change of address): Telephone: 1-800-654-2452 (U.S. and Canada); 314-447-8871 (outside U.S. and Canada). Fax: 314-447-8029. E-mail: journalscustomerservice-usa@elsevier.com (for print support); journalsonlinesupport-usa@elsevier.com (for online support).**

Reprints. For copies of 100 or more, of articles in this publication, please contact the Commercial Reprints Department, Elsevier Inc., 360 Park Avenue South, New York, New York 10010-1710. Tel. 212-633-3874, Fax: 212-633-3820, E-mail: reprints@elsevier.com.

The Surgical Clinics of North America is also published in Spanish by McGraw-Hill Interamericana Editores S.A., P.O. Box 5-237 06500 Mexico D.F. Mexico; and in Portuguese by Interlivros Edicoes Ltda., Rua Comandante Coelho 1085, CEP 21250, Rio de Janeiro, Brazil; and in Greek by Paschalidis Medical Publications, Athens Greece.

The Surgical Clinics of North America is covered in *MEDLINE/PubMed (Index Medicus), EMBASE/Excerpta Medica, Current Contents/Clinical Medicine, Current Contents/Life Sciences, Science Citation Index,* and *ISI/BIOMED.*

Contributors

CONSULTING EDITOR

RONALD F. MARTIN, MD, FACS
Colonel (ret.), United States Army Reserve, Department of Surgery, York Hospital, York, Maine

EDITOR

JUAN M. PALMA-VARGAS
Maine Medical Partners Surgical Care, Portland, Maine

AUTHORS

KAREEM ABU-ELMAGD, MD, PhD, FACS
Professor of Surgery, Cleveland Clinic Lerner College of Medicine, Director, Center for Gut Rehabilitation and Transplantation, Cleveland Clinic, Cleveland, Ohio

SHERIF ARMANYOUS, MD
Research Fellow, Department of Nephrology, Cleveland Clinic, Cleveland, Ohio

BARBRA M. BLAIR, MD
Director, Medical Education for Transplant Infectious Diseases/Immunocompromised Host Program, Department of Medicine, Division of Infectious Diseases, Beth Israel Deaconess Medical Center, Instructor of Medicine, Harvard Medical School, Boston, Massachusetts

DEEPLAXMI BORLE, MD
Abdominal Transplant Surgery Fellow, Department of Surgery, Division of Abdominal Transplant Surgery, Duke University School of Medicine, Durham, North Carolina

GUILHERME COSTA, MD
Staff Surgeon, Center for Gut Rehabilitation and Transplantation, Cleveland Clinic, Cleveland, Ohio

DEV M. DESAI, MD, PhD
Regents Distinguished Scholar in Medical Research, Professor of Surgery and Pediatrics, Chief Pediatric Transplantation, Children's Medical Center, The University of Texas Southwestern Medical Center, Dallas, Texas

STACI A. FISCHER, MD, FACP, FIDSA
Associate Professor of Medicine, The Warren Alpert Medical School of Brown University, Providence, Rhode Island; Employer, Accreditation Council for Graduate Medical Education, Chicago, Illinois

MASATO FUJIKI, MD, PhD
Staff Surgeon, Center for Gut Rehabilitation and Transplantation, Cleveland Clinic, Cleveland, Ohio

CHRISTINE S. HWANG, MD
Associate Professor of Surgery, Children's Medical Center, The University of Texas
Southwestern Medical Center, Dallas, Texas

SAMUEL KESSELI, MD
Resident, Department of Surgery, Duke University Medical Center, Durham,
North Carolina

CHRISTINA L. KLEIN, MD
Medical Director of Kidney and Pancreas Transplantation, Piedmont Transplant Institute,
Piedmont Atlanta Hospital MTP Mason Transplant, Atlanta, Georgia

LUNG-YI LEE, MD
Clinical Instructor, Surgery, Abdominal Transplantation, Stanford University, Stanford,
California

MALCOLM MACCONMARA, MD
Assistant Professor of Surgery, Children's Medical Center, The University of Texas
Southwestern Medical Center, Dallas, Texas

CARLOS E. MARROQUIN, MD, FACS
Chief, Transplant, Immunology and Hepatobiliary Surgery, Department of Surgery,
University of Vermont, Burlington, Vermont

ERIN MAYNARD, MD
Assistant Professor of Surgery, Oregon Health and Science University, Portland, Oregon

MARC L. MELCHER, MD
Associate Professor, Surgery, Abdominal Transplantation, Stanford University, Stanford,
California

MOHAMMED OSMAN, MD
Staff Surgeon, Center for Gut Rehabilitation and Transplantation, Cleveland Clinic,
Cleveland, Ohio

NEHA PAREKH, MS, RD, LD, CNSC
Intestinal Transplant Coordinator, Center for Gut Rehabilitation and Transplantation,
Cleveland Clinic, Cleveland, Ohio

THOMAS A. PHAM, MD
Clinical Assistant Professor, Surgery, Abdominal Transplantation, Stanford University,
Stanford, California

KADIYALA V. RAVINDRA, MBBS
Director, Abdominal Transplant Surgical Fellowship, Associate Professor, Department of
Surgery, Division of Abdominal Transplant Surgery, Duke University School of Medicine,
Durham, North Carolina

ANA P. ROSSI, MD, MPH
Associate Medical Director, Maine Medical Centre, Maine Transplant Program, Portland,
Maine; Clinical Assistant Professor of Medicine, Tufts University, School of Medicine,
Boston, Massachusetts

MARIYA L. SAMOYLOVA, MD, MAS
General Surgery Resident, Department of Surgery, Duke University School of Medicine,
Durham, North Carolina

DEBRA SUDAN, MD
Chief, Division of Abdominal Transplant Surgery, Duke University Medical Center,
Durham, North Carolina

Contents

The incidence of end-stage renal disease has continued to increase. Similarly, the number of patients living with a functioning renal allograft has also increased. Transplantation has improved with advances in surgical techniques, immunosuppression, and better control of comorbid conditions. Transplantation is transformative and offers the greatest potential for restoring a healthy, productive, and durable life to appropriately selected patients. This article describes factors to address in selection of renal transplant candidates and discusses commonly encountered perioperative events. Paramount to selecting appropriate candidates is the collaboration between a multidisciplinary team focused on a systematic process guided by protocols and common practices.

End-stage renal disease (ESRD) is a significant health care burden. Although kidney transplantation is the optimal treatment modality, less than 25% of waiting list patients are transplanted because of organ shortage. Living kidney donation can lead to better recipient and graft survival and increase the number of donors. Not all ESRD patients have potential living donors, and not all living donors are a compatible match to recipients. Kidney paired exchanges allow incompatible pairs to identify compatible living donors for living donor kidney transplants for multiple recipients. Innovative modifications of kidney paired donation can increase the number of kidney transplants, with excellent outcomes.

Posttransplant malignancy is a leading cause of death after solid organ transplantation (SOT). Recipients of SOT are at significantly higher risk of multiple cancers compared with the general population, most notably nonmelanoma skin cancer and posttransplant lymphoproliferative disorders. Risk factors for posttransplant malignancy include history of malignancy, immunosuppression, oncogenic viral infections, sun exposure, and disease-specific associations. Early detection and treatment of malignancies can improve survival.

Liver transplant rates are at an all-time high, with nearly 8000 liver transplants in 2015. Despite the increasing number of liver transplants performed per year, there is a widening gap of supply and demand on limited donor resources. Patient selection is a complex but necessary process to evaluate patients who will benefit from liver transplant while minimizing futile transplants. Efforts should also continue to focus on minimizing perioperative complications resulting in retransplantations and more targeted immunosuppression to minimize side effects and prolong patient survival.

Pediatric liver and kidney transplantation have become the standard and accepted treatment for children with end-stage renal and liver disease. Since the first successful kidney transplant in 1954 by Dr Joseph Murray and the first liver transplant by Dr Thomas Starzl, the scope of indications for visceral organ transplantation as well as the range of recipient and donor ages has expanded. The first pediatric liver and kidney transplants, simultaneous multivisceral transplants, living-donor and donation-after-cardiac-death organs have evolved rapidly into the standard of care for end-stage renal and liver failure in children.

Pancreas transplantation treats insulin-dependent diabetes with or without concurrent end-stage renal disease. Pancreas transplantation increases survival versus no transplant, increases survival when performed as simultaneous pancreas-kidney versus deceased-donor kidney alone, and improves quality of life. Careful donor and recipient selection are paramount to good outcomes. Several technical variations exist for implantation: portal versus systemic vascular drainage and jejunal versus duodenal versus bladder exocrine drainage. Complications are most frequently technical in the first year and immunologic thereafter. Graft rejection is challenging to diagnose and is treated selectively. Islet cell transplantation currently has inferior outcomes to whole-organ pancreas transplantation.

Intestinal and multivisceral transplants are complex technical procedures that present unique challenges in the field of solid organ transplantation. This review aims to highlight the indications, techniques, outcomes, and complications specific to intestinal transplantation.

Infection is an inevitable complication of solid organ transplant. Unrecognized infection may be transmitted from a donor and result in disseminated disease in the immunosuppressed host. Recent outbreaks of deceased donor–derived infections resulting in high rates of mortality and severe morbidity have emphasized the need to be cautious in using donors with possible meningoencephalitis. Screening of organ donors for potential transmissible infections is paramount to improving transplant outcomes.

The successful development of multivisceral and composite visceral transplant is among the milestones in the recent history of human organ transplantation. All types of gastrointestinal transplants have evolved to be the standard of care for patients with gut failure and complex abdominal pathologic conditions. The outcome has markedly improved over the last 3 decades owing to technical innovation, novel immunosuppression, and better postoperative care. Recent data documented significant improvement in the long-term therapeutic indices of all types of visceral transplant close to that achieved with thoracic and solid abdominal organs.

Living safely after organ transplant starts before transplant and continues after transplant. To minimize a solid organ transplant (SOT) recipient's risk for infection and risk for injury, it is important to plan for numerous potential exposures after transplant. These include potential exposure to others with viral or bacterial illness, potential exposure to food and water sources, participation in recreational activities, resuming sexual activity, living with pets, and opportunities for travel, especially internationally. Addressing these risks head-on ensures that SOT recipients and their providers can plan accordingly and anticipate measures that will assist with maintaining such health.

SURGICAL CLINICS
OF NORTH AMERICA

SERIES OF RELATED INTEREST

Advances in Surgery
Available at: www.advancessurgery.com
Surgical Oncology Clinics
Available at: www.surgonc.theclinics.com
Thoracic Surgery Clinics
Available at: www.thoracic.theclinics.com

THE CLINICS ARE AVAILABLE ONLINE!
Access your subscription at:
www.theclinics.com

Foreword

Transplant 2018

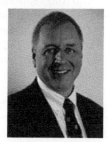

Ronald F Martin, MD, FACS
Consulting Editor

Tribalism has probably existed since there were more than two people. As humans are a subset of social animals, it seems to be their tendency to align with others. It also seems to be a human tendency to define limits to how inclusive these alliances will become. Invariably, there is always a point where "us" ends and "them" begins.

"Us and them," or perhaps more grammatically correct "we and they," have largely been the by-products of the strengths of bonds that could hold groups together. For much of history, those bonds were defined primarily by geographic proximity for the obvious reasons. As our capacity for travel and the ability to influence persons at greater distances became more viable, the bonds of geographic proximity as the main driver for group cohesion became challenged by ideology, religion, central governments, or even the fear of incursion by force as the needs for alliance. Pure local tribalism would be replaced by other forms of tribalism. Also, multiple overlapping allegiances would evolve somewhat by necessity out of these colliding forces of inclusion and exclusion from near and afar.

As we progressed to the modern era with nearly unlimited and decentralized communication, we have become somewhat untethered to local tribal needs in many instances. Much of our original need for local cohesion was to provide common essential needs. Most public services are controlled by laws and regulations making them somewhat immune to tribal force. As such, the basic platforms for safe travel, safe food, safe water, safe commerce, and safe communication are largely secure in many places—but certainly not all places for all of the above. One doesn't have to look too far to find examples of one or more of the above platforms as insecure, but on average, they are secure enough in most circumstances to allow individuals or groups to live in some degree of immediate safety without spending a great deal of

Surg Clin N Am 99 (2019) ix–xi
https://doi.org/10.1016/j.suc.2018.11.001
0039-6109/19/© 2018 Published by Elsevier Inc.

time securing the "home front." A by-product of this safety is allowing most people who wish to the ability to live socially and interpersonally in more "virtual" communities while still having access to the more Malthusian requirements of existence without the personal interrelationships with their geographic neighbors.

Our ability to individually determine with whom we will and won't associate has had a profound effect on our sense of "us" versus "them." Our tribalism has morphed from a need for local cooperation to more ethereal extensions of our beliefs about how the world should be. And, in some instances, to try to deny others their ability to further their beliefs of how the world should be. Furthermore, almost anyone can share their viewpoint in real time with more power than Gutenberg ever dreamed; that is, if one can have their voice heard (or read) above the din of all the other voices.

Our willingness to participate in tribalism is the mechanism by which we define the limits of individualism versus collectivism—somewhere between "going it alone" and "we are all in this together" lives the concept of tribe. We in medicine are not immune to this dilemma and challenge. We are always faced with the competing interests of advocacy. Whether advocating for an individual patient at all costs versus cost containment for all comers or trying to gain competitive advantage for our hospital/ practice versus improving distribution of resources for a larger population, we are all defining tribal boundaries.

I can't think of another group within medicine that has had to wrestle with the issues of tribalism more than our transplant surgery and medicine colleagues. Even within the field it is ironic that for a group that largely tends toward the collectivist end of the spectrum, so much individual effort and sacrifice are demanded. The long and impressive history of the transplant field is littered with broken relationships and personal hardships perhaps more than any other of our disciplines. Even the availability of organs to be transplanted derives from either extreme individual loss or examples of extraordinary generosity or both. Yet, those who are committed to this field have endured and produced amazing advances for not just their patients but for science in general.

Our system of allocating transplant resources (personnel and organs alike) has also tended to the collectivist end of the spectrum as well. As it progressed to the more inclusive models, it has markedly improved its efficiency and the quality of its results in both the short and the long terms. Whether this trend has been a result of altruism, or enlightened self-interest, or perhaps the laws of large numbers, isn't particularly relevant. What matters is that for complex problems with complex and expensive solutions, the collective approach worked better in this instance.

I very much doubt that the transplant model is a reproducible model for most of the clinical challenges we all deal with every day. Still, an understanding of how our colleagues in the transplant world have identified and approached their concerns is very much a beacon of thought that we should all explore. To that end, we are greatly indebted to the contributors to this issue of the *Surgical Clinics of North America* for their insights and wisdom.

Perhaps we should all take inventory of our own tribal views. Perhaps we all consider what the costs of exclusion versus inclusion are or should be. We all wear multiple hats as physicians and surgeons, but that shouldn't imply we can't keep our heads on straight. I hope, as always, that the material we deliver in this series helps you make informed choices for you, your patients, and your communities.

Ronald F. Martin, MD, FACS
Colonel (ret.), United States Army Reserve
Department of Surgery
York Hospital
16 Hospital Drive, Suite A
York, ME 03909, USA

E-mail address:
rmartin@yorkhospital.com

Patient Selection for Kidney Transplant

Carlos E. Marroquin, MD

KEYWORDS

- Kidney transplant • End-stage renal disease • Renal-replacement therapy
- Patient selection

KEY POINTS

- The incidence of end-stage renal disease (ESRD) has increased steadily over the last several decades.
- There have been dramatic improvements in the outcomes following transplantation with a significant increase in the number of patients receiving renal-replacement therapy in the form of a transplant.
- Transplantation is transformative and offers the greatest potential for restoring a healthy, productive, and durable life to appropriately selected patients.

The incidence of end-stage renal disease (ESRD) has increased steadily over the last several decades, in part because of the obesity epidemic, alone or in combination with an increased incidence of diabetes, and hypertension. As a result, the number of patients who receive treatment of ESRD has increased significantly over the last three decades. Most receive renal-replacement therapy in the form of dialysis. Alternatively, some of these patients receive renal-replacement therapy in the form of transplantation. Similar to the growth in the ESRD and dialysis population, the number of patients receiving renal-replacement therapy in the form of a transplant has also grown. This is because of advances in surgical technique, improvements in immunosuppression, and better control of associated comorbid conditions. Despite advances in the treatment of patients with ESRD, kidney transplantation is transformative and offers the greatest potential for restoring a healthy, productive, and durable life to appropriately selected patients. This article describes factors that should be addressed in the selection of renal transplant candidates and discusses commonly encountered perioperative events. Paramount to the process of selecting appropriate candidates is the collaborative interactions of a multidisciplinary team focused on a systematic and

The author has nothing to disclose.
Transplant, Immunology and Hepatobiliary Surgery, Department of Surgery, University of Vermont, 111 Colchester Avenue, Burlington, VT 05401, USA
E-mail address: carlos.marroquin@uvmhealth.org

Surg Clin N Am 99 (2019) 1–35
https://doi.org/10.1016/j.suc.2018.09.002

expeditious process guided by protocols and common practices from the moment a patient presents with ESRD.

Patients with kidney disease may present with a variety of complaints. Some patients manifest extrarenal signs of kidney disease, such as swelling, nausea, vomiting, confusion, and lethargy. In the extreme, patients may develop severe metabolic derangements, pericardial effusions, and congestive heart failure. These are all signs of uremia and progressive renal dysfunction. Other patients have obvious signs of kidney injury, such as hematuria, and flank pain, and another group of patients are completely asymptomatic but are found to have high blood pressure, elevated serum creatinine, or an abnormal urinalysis during a routine examination. Once kidney disease is suspected, one must establish the cause of the renal disease. This begins with a thorough history and physical examination. Useful studies in the evaluation of kidney disease include a urinalysis, measurement of urinary protein excretion, and an ultrasound. Although underused, kidney biopsies serve to provide a histologic diagnosis. However, biopsies are often confounded by the presence of severe fibrosis because most patients have advanced renal injury that is manifested histologically by nonspecific fibrosis.

The next step in the evaluation of a patient with kidney disease is to establish the extent of the disease. A serum creatinine is an inaccurate surrogate of renal function. The glomerular filtration rate (GFR) allows one to establish the degree of renal injury and to follow the course of the disease. The normal value for GFR depends on age, sex, and body size. Kidney function tends to decline with age and by 65 years of age, most everyone has some degree of kidney disease. A decrease in GFR suggests progression of the underlying disease or the development of a superimposed disease.

Chronic kidney disease is broken down into five stages (**Table 1**), with each stage being defined by the GFR and progressive levels of renal injury. Although there are more accurate methods of measuring GFR, such as inulin excretion, radioactive iothalamate, and sodium iothalamate, the GFR is estimated from the Modification of Diet in Renal Disease (MDRD) Study equation, which takes into account the serum creatinine and other variables known to affect overall renal function, such as age, gender, race, and body size.[1,2] The MDRD equation uses creatinine values with age, gender, and race to estimate the GFR. This formula is normalized to an average adult body surface area of 1.73 m². As such, it does not require measures for height or weight.

Any patient with ESRD should be considered as a potential transplant candidate. In fact, it is a federal regulation that all patients who initiate dialysis be considered for referral to a transplant center for evaluation of transplant candidacy. However, if they do not meet the transplant center's written minimal criteria (eg, they have known malignancy, or known cardiovascular disease with an ejection fraction of <40%), they

Table 1
Five stages of chronic kidney disease

Stage	Description	GFR (mL/min/1.73 m²)
1	Kidney damage with normal GFR	90
2	Kidney damage with mild GFR	60–89
3	Kidney damage with moderate GFR	30–59
4	Kidney damage with severe GFR	15–29
5	Kidney failure	<15

GFR (mL/min/1.73 m²) = 175 × SCr (exp[-1.154]) × age (exp[-0.203]) × (0.742 if female) × (1.21 if African American). Scr, serum creatinine.

do not need to be formally evaluated at the center. The criteria do need to be documented supporting the decision not to refer for transplant evaluation. Although renal failure from diabetes and glomerulonephritis are the most common indications for transplantation, the causes of ESRD and indications for transplantation are multiple. **Box 1** lists many of the causes of renal disease and indications for transplantation.

Because of the kidney entitlement portion of the Social Security Amendments of The Medicare Disability Act of 1972, all US citizens with ESRD have their dialysis costs paid for by Medicare.[3] As such, it is a Medicare requirement that all patients requiring dialysis in the United States be given the option to be evaluated for renal transplantation because it has been shown to be less morbid and more cost effective to transplant patients rather than remaining on life-long hemodialysis. Moreover, transplantation significantly reduces the morbidity and mortality of patients who remain on the waitlist when compared with age-matched cohorts who remain on dialysis. It is important to keep in mind that many patients do not meet minimum criteria for transplantation, and comparing these patients to transplant recipients gives a less accurate view of the benefits of transplantation. There is clearly a greater annual mortality for patients with ESRD on hemodialysis. This annual mortality is lower for patients who are deemed to be transplant candidates and listed and is reduced most for patients who undergo transplant and have a functioning renal allograft.[4] Every 12 months, all patients undergoing dialysis should be re-evaluated by their nephrologist, and those who meet their local transplant center's criteria should be referred for transplant evaluation.

It is critical to perform the pretransplant evaluation in a systematic manner to ensure candidates are properly selected to maximize the use of a scarce resource, the renal allograft, and the post-transplant patient and allograft survival while minimizing potential pain and suffering. Transplantation is the only field in medicine that truly changes the natural history of disease and offers patients and their families the gift of life. The real challenge transplant programs face is the huge disparity between organ supply and demand. In 2017, there were 19,850 kidney transplants performed of 95,105 candidates.[5] Americans are living longer and more patients are being added to the waitlist as new candidates. In addition, some candidates are being listed for the second, third, and fourth transplant. As such, the demand has far outpaced the supply.

Transplant professionals cannot simply rely on an evaluation of a given patient's surgical candidacy, but also need to thoroughly evaluate a candidate's ability to engage in behavioral modifications that help them live a healthy lifestyle to improve their survival. This is critical because transplant candidates and recipients have many socioeconomic barriers and multiple medical comorbidities that evolve and are often associated with their end-organ disease. As such, it is key to mitigate these barriers and comorbidities that may potentially threaten the lifespan and quality of the transplanted organ and transplant recipient. To this end, patients must undergo a thorough evaluation before being listed for a potential transplant. The evaluation process involves a multidisciplinary group of professionals starting with a cursory screening process with a transplant coordinator. The initial screening process should evaluate programmatic inclusion criteria and absolute and relative exclusion criteria. Although every program has variations of each, there are generally accepted criteria that most transplant programs believe are critical.[6] Transplantation is resource intensive. As such, programs need to partner with a variety of other health care providers to develop protocols and practices. Programs need to adhere to the protocols and practices they create with the intent to evaluate their processes with regularity with the objective of continual improvement.

Box 1
Indications for renal transplant

Congenital disorders
  Renal aplasia
  Hypoplasia
  Horseshoe kidney

Toxic nephropathies
  Lead nephropathy
  Analgesic nephropathy

Irreversible acute renal failure
  Cortical necrosis
  Hemolytic uremic syndrome
  Acute and subacute glomerulonephritis
  Anaphylactoid purpura (Henoch-Schönlein)
  Acute tubular necrosis

Metabolic disorders
  Hyperoxaluria
  Nephrocalcinosis
  Gout
  Oxalosis
  Amyloidosis
  Cytinosis

Tumors requiring nephrectomy
  Renal cell carcinoma
  Wilms tumor
  Tuberous sclerosis

Hereditary nephropathies
  Alport syndrome
  Polycystic kidney disease
  Medullary cystic disease

Obstructive uropathies
  Acquired
  Congenital

Irreversible chronic renal failure
  Chronic pyelonephritis
  Chronic glomerulonephritis
  Diabetic nephropathy
  Goodpasture syndrome
  Hypocomplementemic nephritis
  Hypertensive nephrosclerosis

Other causes of renal failure
  Multiple myeloma
  Macroglobulinemia
  Wegener disease
  Scleroderma systemic lupus
  Erythematosis
  Polyarteritis nodosa

Trauma requiring nephrectomy

SELECTION CRITERIA

Transplant candidates must have documented chronic renal disease defined by GFR less than 20 or they must be on some form of renal-replacement therapy consisting of hemodialysis or peritoneal dialysis. This is the only hard inclusion criteria for candidacy. Although there is one single inclusion criteria, the number of exclusionary criteria vary from program to program. The goal of the evaluation is to be certain patients are physically, emotionally, and financially ready to get through a transplant and enjoy a long post-transplant survival with little to no harm following the transplant. The evaluation can vary depending on the structure and programmatic resources, but all potential transplant candidates require a thorough evaluation[6] and education by a transplant dietitian, transplant pharmacist, transplant financial coordinator, transplant social worker, transplant nephrologist, and surgeon.

The nephrologist and surgeon evaluate patients for medical issues that would present contraindications to renal transplantation. All patients are evaluated thoroughly looking for comorbid conditions that would affect their surgical candidacy and complicate the transplant outcome. Medical risk factors for cardiac disease, pulmonary disease, peripheral vascular disease, and infectious issues are some of the factors that are evaluated. Findings on physical examination guide further studies and consultations. Patients at risk have noninvasive cardiac studies, lower extremity and carotid testing, followed by invasive testing and referral to the vascular service before listing if indicated. In addition to a global evaluation, certain circumstances must be addressed specifically because the goal is to improve each candidate's life, in terms of duration and quality, without inducing unnecessary pain and suffering.

AGE

There is no universal agreement on what age, if any, should be excluded for transplantation. Historically, the transplant community defined older recipients as being 60 to 65. As such, there is a paucity of data evaluating the outcomes of transplanting patients older than 65. Although Rao and coworkers[7] demonstrated a survival advantage in recipients older than 70, not all studies have found transplantation to confer a survival benefit in this elderly group. Wolfe and colleagues[4] demonstrated that the cumulative survival rate improved following the first year after transplantation among patients who were 60 to 74. When this subgroup was further subdivided into patients who were 60 to 64 years of age, 65 to 69 years of age, and those who were 70 to 74 years of age, the projected increases in the life span were 4.3 years, 2.8 years, and 1.0 year, respectively. This suggests a diminishing return for the older group of recipients.

Our group identified and studied primary renal transplant recipients from 1988 to 2014 in the United Network of Organ Sharing database and found elderly renal transplant recipients experience lower graft survival rates and were at increased risk for graft loss from primary nonfunction and infection. We also found they had lower risk of loss from recurrent disease and rejection than younger recipients (unpublished data). The implications for clinical care are numerous. Paramount among these implications is the notion that a transplant may not be in the best interest of these patients.

Septuagenarians, candidates between the ages of 70 and 79, who are referred for transplantation are usually the healthiest 70 year olds on hemodialysis. We must appreciate that we can substantially alter their "healthy life" at the time of referral with an attempted invasive procedure, such as a kidney transplant. Although they may tolerate the procedure, the addition of immunosuppressive medications further complicates the recovery from surgery and long-term outcomes. The risks may be much greater in any 70 year old's case than the marginal benefit from a transplant. When one considers that the natural lifespan of Americans is 81 for healthy women and 76 for healthy men, there is a greater likelihood one would negatively impact that natural lifespan than improve their last decade.

Older age, in association with other existing conditions, such as ESRD, heart disease, diabetes, and hypertension, increases the risk of complications. These complications, in turn, increase the rate of delayed graft function and many other postoperative events including infectious and cardiovascular complications that result in a prolonged hospitalization and even death. In fact, older age is known to be an independent risk factor for the development of delayed graft function that may result in graft loss.[8] Moreover, elderly recipients are known to have lower survival rates. It is known that older patients are more prone to complications after most procedures, and these complications are aggravated in patients with ESRD and the need for post-transplant immunosuppressive medications. As such, we caution that patients older than 70 years of age need to be approached with a great deal of judgment because one could significantly alter their survival and well-being.

FRAILTY

Frailty affects perioperative outcomes, long-term outcomes, and postoperative mortality. Frailty is likely a factor that contributes to some of the poor outcomes observed in older transplant recipients. Moreover, because ESRD can inflict a progressive deterioration to one's health and reserve, patients with end-organ disease may often be young patients being evaluated but have had many years of concomitant end-organ disease with associated multisystem morbidities. These multiple comorbidities contribute to overall lack of well-being and/or frailty. Although it is reasonably easy to select healthy patients who will benefit from a renal transplant, the challenge is in identifying individuals who would be harmed by going through a transplant and distinguish them from those who would benefit from preconditioning. Transplant programs should incorporate a mechanism to reliably identify frailty that can be applied with facility and regularity to allow early identification of candidates at risk and allow comparisons over time.

One of the components of frailty is physical reserve that is affected by physical strength and fitness. Mobility and balance are surrogates of physical strength, which is measured by the short physical performance battery[9–12] at a single point in time, and is predictive of all-cause mortality, but fails to capture potential decline in strength and endurance over time. The Fried Frailty Assessment provides a more global evaluation of fitness and reserve and has been validated in patients with ESRD[13–15] before and after transplantation.

Because frailty is affected by more than simply "physical fitness," an objective measure of nutritional status is an important tool to assessing frailty. The Malnutrition Inflammation Score has been studied in a comparison of eight different nutrition-related tests to predict mortality in hemodialysis patients[16] and was found to be predictive of mortality. Moreover, it was also found to be predictive of an increased risk of cardiovascular events and infections. Because two of the leading causes of death with a functioning renal allograft are cardiovascular events and infections, adopting the Malnutrition Inflammation Score to assess nutritional status in the context of its ability to predict mortality, cardiovascular events, and infections in hemodialysis patients may prove useful in kidney transplant patients. Given its predictive nature, patients who are found to be frail should not proceed to listing or transplant until they improve their state of frailty with preconditioning.

BODY MASS INDEX

Increasing body mass index places recipients at increased risk of complications that translate into poor outcomes with the potential of ending with graft loss.[17] Kidney transplant recipients who are obese have been found to experience more complications, such as infection, wound dehiscence, evisceration, ventral hernia, allograft failure, gangrene, necrotizing fasciitis, postoperative bleeding, and intra-abdominal infections. They also require repeated surgeries and have a greater risk of death. They are also at risk of specific post-transplant-related complications consisting of greater risk of biopsy-proven rejection, greater rates of delayed graft function, and allograft loss.[18] Because these complications are found in greater frequency in the overweight population, transplant candidates with body mass index greater than 38 should be counseled to participate in medically supervised weight loss programs before being listed for a potential transplant.

PSYCHOSOCIAL, FINANCIAL, AND PERSONAL SUPPORT SYSTEM

The transplant social worker, transplant financial counselor, transplant pharmacist, and transplant nurse coordinator evaluate patients' support system, insurance, financial status, and psychosocial issues that may contraindicate transplantation. Inadequate health insurance coverage for kidney transplant and/or prescribed medications could result in significant economic hardship and inability to obtain necessary medications would compromise the transplant outcome and potentially the recipient's well-being and life. Programs should evaluate the adequacy of insurance coverage and should provide counseling regarding coverage and anticipated expenses at the time of initial screening, and should not invite the candidate to begin their evaluation until adequate insurance is verified. Verifying adequate coverage is important to prevent the process from moving forward with a patient who is ultimately unable to be listed either because of inadequate coverage or because of denial by their insurance carrier.

All patients are counseled regarding their need for life-long immunosuppressive medication, and the substantial cost of these medications. Because most patients are Medicare eligible, 80% of their post-transplant immunosuppressive medications are covered. Patients younger than 65 years of age have immunosuppressive coverage for a minimum of 3 years. These young recipients lose Medicare coverage 3 years after their transplant unless they have another Medicare-qualifying condition. This coverage does not include nonimmunosuppressive medications, such as prophylactic antimicrobial agents, and these must be paid for out-of-pocket or from another source of coverage. Patients who are unable to afford their medications cannot and should not be transplanted because medical noncompliance, for any reason, results in complications that not only risk poor allograft survival, but also jeopardize patient survival. Patients are also counseled regarding medical interactions and a multitude of risks and side effects of immunosuppressive medications for the first time by a transplant pharmacist.

Transplant candidates are also evaluated for a history of repeated noncompliance with prescribed medical therapies through evaluation of their dialysis history and medical history. Candidates who have obvious noncompliance documented and identified during their initial screening should be counseled and turned away until the behavioral issues clearly improve. In a similar fashion, transplant candidates are evaluated for a history of drug and/or alcohol misuse. These potential transplant candidates may be rereferred once evidence of compliance is established. Finally, patients who are unable to participate in their own care because of other conditions (ie, dementia, Down syndrome) and have no effective support would not do well post-transplant and may fair better with an alternate form of renal-replacement therapy until adequate support is demonstrated. Patients with ESRD in need of a transplant present with

Table 2
Screening guidelines for malignancy

Malignancy	Screening
Cervical cancer	Pelvic examination with Papanicolaou testing (1–3 y in women 20–65 who have a cervix)
Uterine cancer	Pelvic examination with Papanicolaou testing (1–3 y in women 20–65 who have a cervix)
Testicular cancer	Testicular examination during evaluation
Kaposi sarcoma (increased risk in African and Middle East origin, hepatitis B infection, prior history or family history of Kaposi sarcoma, and men who have sex with men)	Human herpes virus-8 antibodies
Breast cancer	Breast self-examination monthly beginning at age 20 Breast examination with evaluation for transplant Annual mammogram beginning at age 40 Women with family history of breast cancer in first-degree relative should have their first mammogram 10 y earlier than the age of onset of breast cancer in their relative
Colorectal cancer	Colonoscopy starting at 50 Earlier for high-risk candidates based on personal and family history
Prostate cancer	Digital rectal examination and prostate-specific antigen starting at age 50
Liver cancer	Ultrasound of liver in high-risk groups (hepatitis B and C positive)
Lung cancer	Low-dose computed tomography

significant social and economic factors that need to be evaluated and alleviated before listing. Programmatic processes to assist patients negotiate some or all of these social and financial factors are critical to make them good transplant candidates.

CANCER

Patients with ESRD on renal-replacement therapy are known to have a greater incidence of cancer.[19] Once transplanted, immunosuppression increases this risk substantially by inhibiting the immune surveillance of cancers and oncogenic viruses. As such, patients should undergo standardized evaluation for malignancy before being transplanted. This evaluation should involve standard screening (**Table 2**) and take into consideration patient-specific risk factors based on personal and family history and should follow the American Cancer Society Guidelines for screening.[20] Patients with rare syndromic etiologies of ESRD should have a genetic evaluation to establish risk of associated malignancies with appropriate screening.

It is also critical to establish any prior history of malignancy. Patients with a history of prior malignancy should be evaluated by a medical oncologist before moving forward with an evaluation. The patient's oncologist should be consulted and requested to provide a clear opinion on the patient's prognosis, the risk of recurrence, and any foreseeable issues or concerns following transplantation. Moreover, a recommended surveillance should be outlined and completed before listing and/or undergoing a transplant to avoid the ravages of recurrent disease. We have learned from the Israel Penn Tumor Registry at the University of Cincinnati that patients who undergo transplant early after completing their tumor treatment experience a greater recurrence rate than those patients who are transplanted later after completing their therapy.[21] Therefore, candidates with a history of malignancy should not be invited to begin their evaluation until a recommended surveillance period has been completed (**Table 3**). Finally, a thorough evaluation with physical examination, and appropriate diagnostic and imaging studies should be performed to confirm the absence of recurrence before listing.

INFECTIONS

Programs should work to elicit a history of infections to ensure proper therapy has been provided and to establish proper prophylaxis following transplantation. In addition to a thorough history of past infections, programs should inquire if patients have lived in areas known to be endemic for certain infectious pathogens. This is critical information to obtain because immunosuppressive medications following transplantation increase the risk of recurrence or activation. Certain fungal infections are endemic to specific regions of the United States and transplant candidates who live or have lived in these regions are at risk. Histoplasmosis is the most common endemic

Table 3
Guidelines for candidates wait time following a diagnosis and treatment of cancer

Malignancy	Minimum Wait Time
Renal cell carcinoma	Symptomatic <5 cm = 2 y Symptomatic >5 cm = 5 y Incidental with no capsular penetration = none
Bladder cancer	Invasive bladder cancer = 2 y In situ noninvasive = none
Cervical cancer	Low grade = 2 y All others = 5 y
Uterine body	2 y
Testicular cancer	2 y
Thyroid cancer	2 y
Sarcoma	5 y
Breast cancer	5 y
Colorectal cancer	5 y
Prostate cancer	2 y
Hepatocellular cancer	6 mo following full recovery from liver transplant for hepatocellular carcinoma
Multiple myeloma	Contraindication to transplant
Lymphomas	2–5 y
Leukemias	2 y
Skin cancer	Basal cell = none Localized squamous cell = 2 y Malignant melanoma = 5 y Merkel cell carcinoma = 5 y
Lung cancer	2 y
Neuroendocrine malignancies	5 y

mycosis and afflicts the Southeast and Midwest. Coccidioidomycosis is endemic to western states. Blastomycosis, the least prevalent, is commonly found in Midwestern states.[22] The physical examination is critical to assess active infectious processes affecting transplant candidates. Patients on peritoneal dialysis are prone to secondary bacterial peritonitis and should be examined for signs of infection. If concerned, a fluid sample should be sent to the laboratory for cell count and Gram stain with cultures. Patients with diabetes are prone to peripheral vascular disease and need to be examined looking for signs of active infection, and ulceration. A history of claudication or rest pain should prompt a vascular consultation for further evaluation and assessment for revascularization. Patients who develop osteomyelitis require definitive therapy and proof of resolution before being listed. These patients should not be considered for transplantation until their active infectious risks are resolved.

Active or unresolved infections must be resolved before listing. If a given patient has been listed and subsequently develops an infection, they should be inactivated until they are re-evaluated to be certain the infection has been effectively treated and cleared. Candidates who are transplanted with an active infection are at risk of developing uncontrollable sequelae of their infection and could progress to sepsis and death as a result of needed immunosuppression. Some infections may require long-term therapy before consideration should be given to listing and transplanting. Although programs cannot screen for all possible infectious pathogens, every effort should be made to screen for prevalent organisms known to afflict dialysis patients and known to increase the morbidity and mortality following a transplant and administration of immunosuppressive medications (**Box 2**).

One of the sequelae of human immunodeficiency virus (HIV) infection includes nephropathy and some of these patients go on to develop ESRD. The prevalence of chronic kidney disease in the HIV-infected populations ranges from 2% to 38%[23] depending on geographic region. Since the advent of highly active antiretroviral therapy, the survival of HIV-positive patients has improved. In fact, HIV has become a chronic disease and patients are going on to develop chronic diseases afflicting the general aging population. ESRD not uncommonly results with demand for renal-replacement therapy in the form of hemodialysis, and peritoneal dialysis. HIV infection is not uncommon in the dialysis population with a reported incidence varying from 0.3% to 2.6% of dialysis patients.[24]

In otherwise healthy HIV-positive patients, transplantation is rapidly becoming a viable means of renal-replacement therapy. Transplants in HIV-positive candidates are being performed at a small number of programs with good results.[25,26] This endeavor requires highly specialized multidisciplinary collaboration because specialized knowledge of antiretroviral regimens, drug interactions, HIV pathophysiology, immunosuppression, and post-transplant sequelae are necessary to care

---

Box 2
Common organisms affecting dialysis and transplant patients

Human immunodeficiency virus

Tuberculosis

Hepatitis B and C

Cytomegalovirus

Epstein-Barr virus

Human T-lymphotropic virus 1 and 2

for this patient population. The general consensus is that HIV-positive transplant candidates should have an undetectable viral load and a CD4 count greater than 250 before referral. These candidates are also expected to meet all other center-specific criteria to be listed (ie, no evidence of malignancy, specifically Kaposi sarcoma).

The incidence of tuberculosis (TB) in the dialysis population is much greater than TB in the general population,[27] and these patients are more likely to develop TB than the general population. In these patients, the diagnosis of TB disease is often difficult. Patients with ESRD on dialysis are often malnourished and immunosuppressed, which makes them anergic. As such, the classic tuberculin skin test has a low sensitivity and not an insignificant specificity in people who received the bacille Calmette-Guérin vaccine.[28] However, screening is critical to decrease or prevent reactivation and broad dissemination with immunosuppression. Moreover, patients who develop TB following renal transplant demonstrated significant allograft dysfunction.[29] Screening should be performed with one of any of the interferon-γ release assays because they have superior sensitivity and specificity for the diagnosis of TB compared with the tuberculin skin test.[30] Patients who test positive should be referred to an infectious disease specialist for treatment and should only be listed for transplant after completing an adequate course of therapy.

Hepatitis C virus (HCV) infection is not uncommon in patients on hemodialysis.[31,32] As such, kidney transplant candidates should be tested for anti-HCV antibodies. If anti-HCV antibodies are present, then the candidate has had an exposure to HCV and should have a quantitative test for HCV RNA. Historically, efforts to clear HCV before transplantation were met with poor results and were also associated with a variety of treatment-related complications to include rejection and allograft loss as a result of interferon-based therapies.[32] The new era of direct-acting antiviral agents is changing this landscape.[33,34] Although these new therapies are capable of eradicating HCV, there is growing support for delaying therapy until after transplantation. This would have the advantage of a quicker time to transplant by increasing the donor pool to HCV-positive donors. Once transplanted, recipients known to be HCV-positive and those receiving an HCV-positive kidney should initiate treatment after a period of stability to avoid potential injuries to the allograft.

Despite a clear decline in the incidence of hepatitis B virus (HBV) infections in the general population as a result of routine vaccination, HBV infections are more common in patients with ESRD on hemodialysis. Transplant candidates should be screened with three HBV screening serum markers: (1) hepatitis B surface antigen, (2) antibody to hepatitis B surface antigen, and (3) antibody to hepatitis B core antigen.[35] Patients found to be positive for hepatitis B surface antigen and/or hepatitis B core antigen should have a hepatitis B DNA assay to measure the quantity of HBV. Patients who have been vaccinated successfully have antibody to hepatitis B surface antigen levels and therefore are not necessarily infected. We recommend patients who are found to be infected with HBV be referred for consultation with an infectious disease provider or hepatologist to evaluate and initiate therapy. We also recommend engaging the consultant to discuss initiating pretransplant treatment with antiviral therapy and establishing a plan for post-transplant therapy. We believe strongly that treatment is critical and is needed long-term because there are many reports of fatal reactivation following withdrawal of therapy in immunosuppressed patients.[36,37] HBV DNA can re-emerge as a result of active immunosuppression leading to progressive liver injury culminating in death. As such, antiviral therapy should be combined with periodic liver function testing and quantitative measurements of HBV DNA.

Chronic HCV and HBV infections are not uncommon in the dialysis population and important causes of morbidity and mortality in renal transplant recipients. Therefore, candidates need to be evaluated and all candidates who test positive for either HCV or HBV should have imaging studies and a transjugular or percutaneous liver biopsy performed. Those candidates with evidence of cirrhosis with active viral infection should be considered a relative contraindication to transplantation and must meet minimum criteria (**Box 3**), because their survival may be shortened by the necessary immunosuppression.

There are other viruses for which we recommend testing. Although these do not represent a contraindication to proceeding with listing or a transplant, they can emerge as significant pathogens because they can produce substantial morbidity and require a planned approach. Cytomegalovirus (CMV) is a lymphotropic DNA virus that is a member of the herpes virus family. CMV is spread by person-to-person contact and through solid organ transplantation when the donor was previously infected. CMV is prevalent in the general population. Although almost everyone is infected with this virus, it is not pathologic in an immune-competent host. There are well-established protocols for managing CMV and they are based on risk factors for CMV infections. Once a person is infected with CMV (primary infection), the virus becomes latent in white blood cells. As such, donors, cadaveric and living, who have been previously infected with CMV are able to transmit CMV infection.

Donor-to-recipient mismatch status, that is, a donor who is known to be CMV-positive to a recipient who is CMV-negative, is the most common and well-identified risk factor for developing a CMV infection. Another risk factor is the extent of immunosuppression. Recipients who receive induction with anti-thymocyte globulin or alemtuzumab are considered at high risk of reactivation of CMV because of the strength of induction immunosuppression. These patients generally receive prophylaxis with an antiviral agent, such as valganciclovir, for anywhere from 3 to 6 months depending on the programmatic protocol. Allograft rejection is another well-established risk factor because the treatment of rejection generally requires augmentation in the amount of immunosuppression thereby increasing the risk of reactivation. The risk of CMV disease depends on the interaction of all known risk factors to include many host-dependent factors, such as the recipient's nutritional status, immune competence (innate and adaptive immunity), and degree of conditioning, all of which contribute to the patient's overall risk when combined with the extent of immunosuppression.

CMV infection is inconsequential in an immune-competent host. As such, we cannot underscore the role of immunosuppressive therapy as a risk factor. The strength of

---

Box 3
Chronic active hepatitis B/C: minimum criteria for listing

- No evidence of cirrhosis on liver biopsy
- No evidence of hepatocellular carcinoma on imaging
- Needs to be actively followed by hepatology
- Needs to be adherent with regimen (HBV)
- Hepatitis B viremia needs to be controlled with therapy
  - HBV (lamivudine/adefovir/entecavir)
- Consider treatment following transplantation

induction immunosuppression and degree of maintenance immunosuppression are two pharmacologic means of increasing risk of infection. Because of the global nature of immunosuppression, other associated factors include coinfections with other viruses, bacteria, and opportunistic fungal infections. As such, conversion in a given patient's CMV status post-transplant should also prompt providers to look for other opportunistic infections because conversion in CMV status speaks to a significant degree of immune-compromised state and increased risk for infectious complications. All transplant candidates should be screened for a history of CMV infection with antibody assays. It is recommended that those candidates found to be CMV naive who are recipients of a CMV-positive allograft and those recipients who receive powerful induction therapy, regardless of CMV status, should receive antiviral prophylaxis. The risk/benefit of prophylaxis versus expectant observation has biologic and financial costs to the patient. The approach is one that must be determined by each program as the risk and benefit of reactivation versus costs are assessed.

Epstein-Barr virus (EBV) is another virus that can produce substantial morbidity after a solid organ transplant (SOT) and requires a planned approach to include knowledge of serum status before transplantation. EBV is also a member of the herpes virus family, and also prevalent in adults. The incidence of infections with EBV increases as humans age. EBV spreads through bodily fluids with saliva being a common source of transmission accounting for infectious mononucleosis in teenagers. Once a given person is infected, they develop antibodies against EBV that becomes protective and a means of verifying previous infection. EBV infects B cells of the immune system and once the initial EBV infection is cleared, the EBV virus can lie dormant in the immune system's B cells for life.[38]

EBV-negative recipients of EBV-positive organs and EBV-positive recipients are at greater risk of developing post-transplant lymphoproliferative disorder (PTLD) following induction immunosuppression. Again, the strength of induction immunosuppression and degree of maintenance immunosuppression are two pharmacologic means of increasing the risk of developing PTLD with childhood recipients of SOTs being affected the most, likely because they tend to receive aggressive immunosuppressive regimens. PTLDs are a type of lymphoma that involve uncontrolled proliferation of lymphoid cells as a consequence of immunosuppression after SOT or hematopoietic stem cell transplant.[39] PTLD induces substantial morbidity with potential allograft loss and not insignificant mortality.

VACCINATIONS

Once transplanted, the risk of infectious complications increases substantially because of the necessity to take immunosuppressive medications. This is often compounded in patients with end-organ disease and malnutrition who start out in an immune-compromised state. Some infections may be prevented with pretransplant vaccination. Transplant candidates should have their immunization history reviewed and updated before they are transplanted (**Box 4**).[40] Live vaccines should never be administered to a transplant recipient who is being actively immunosuppressed. Therefore, it is strongly recommended to administer live vaccines, such as mumps, measles, rubella, varicella, and zoster vaccines before being listed for a transplant. Although pretransplant vaccination early in the course of the evaluation should be the standard, inactivated vaccines are safe following transplantation but should not be given within 6 months of a transplant because the benefits are attenuated by the degree of immunosuppression that is commonly greatest during this early period.

Box 4
Vaccines recommended before transplant listing
Influenza
Hepatitis A and B
Tetanus
Pertussis
Inactivated polio
Streptococcus pneumoniae
Neisseria meningitides
Rabies
Human papilloma virus
Mumps, measles, rubella
Varicella
BCG

DENTAL EXAMINATION

Dental infections are a potential source of morbidity and in the extreme, as in Ludwig angina, potentially lethal for transplant candidates. As such, all transplant candidates should be evaluated during their initial and annual wait-list examinations. All patients should be seen by a dentist for dental and oral health clearance, but the patient's oral hygiene should be assessed even once cleared. If any signs of infection of either the teeth or gums is evident, then they should not proceed with evaluation or should be inactivated until the candidate is evaluated and cleared by a dentist.

TOBACCO/NICOTINE PRODUCT USE

Smoking tobacco increases the risk of morbidity and mortality in the general population and is a substantial health risk for kidney transplant recipients because it is associated with lung cancer, heart disease, peripheral vascular disease, and graft loss. Transplant recipients who continued smoking after transplant had a greater than 100% increased risk of noncardiovascular death, 70% greater risk of all-cause mortality, and a 50% greater risk of graft loss.[41] This increased risk was not seen in transplant recipients who were former smokers. Even receiving a renal transplant from a smoker donor increases the risk of death for the recipient and carries a poorer graft survival compared with nonsmoking donors.[42] As such, a strong emphasis should be placed on smoking cessation before kidney transplantation.

CARDIAC EVALUATION

Patients with ESRD are at high risk of cardiovascular disease. In fact, the day a given patient is diagnosed with ESRD, one can assume that patient has started evolving heart disease. The progressive decrease in renal function leads to disturbances of mineral metabolism that leads to secondary hyperparathyroidism. This results in an association between ESRD and a disorder of mineral and bone metabolism that leads to vascular calcification.[43] As such, there is a tight association between vascular disorders and chronic kidney disease. As patients lose nephron function, uremia induces an oxidative stress and abnormalities in calcium metabolism that result in calcium deposition in arterial intima with subsequent loss of arterial compliance as atherosclerosis evolves. The end result is an increased incidence of myocardial infarctions in patients with ESRD. Vascular insults are compounded by the association of diabetes and hypertension with ESRD.

In addition to vascular insults, chronic renal dysfunction may lead to heart failure.[44] This should be viewed as an inevitable relationship because the same risk factors that contribute to the onset of renal disease (diabetes, obesity, and hypertension) are critical to the development of heart failure. Death from myocardial infarction and arrhythmia are the largest causes of noninfectious death in renal transplant recipients. Cardiovascular morbidity and mortality are particularly high in the perioperative period after a kidney transplant. As such, it is critical to screen transplant candidates for cardiovascular disease to ensure safe and effective kidney transplantation can occur. The cardiac criteria for evaluating potential renal transplant recipients need to be more critical than the criteria developed for routine cardiac clearance for noncardiac surgical procedures by the American Society of Cardiology. Moreover, every kidney transplant program should develop an association with a cardiology group that can help sort out cardiovascular risk in this high-risk population.

All patients should have an electrocardiogram (EKG) and echocardiogram as part of the initial intake to the kidney transplant program. If the transplant candidate has no prior cardiac history and is younger than 40 years of age, the echocardiogram and EKG should be updated every 2 years. Echocardiograms should be repeated annually in patients with valvular defects that are moderate or severe, and in patients found to have left ventricular ejection fraction less than 50%, or pulmonary artery pressure estimate of greater than 40 mm Hg. Because it is known that patients with progressive renal disease are at greater than average risk of coronary artery disease (CAD), cardiac stress testing should be a staple in the evaluation of a potential kidney transplant recipient. Because developing ESRD initiates a cascade of events that affects the coronary vasculature and because initiating dialysis produces a second biologic stressor to the coronaries and time on dialysis has been shown to be a risk factor for CAD,[45] all patients with at least 2 years dialysis, regardless of age, should undergo cardiac imaging stress test every 2 years. Candidates between the ages of 40 and 60 require cardiac stress test as part of the initial intake if they have two or more risk factors for CAD (**Box 5**).

Some candidates present with a known history of CAD or have inordinate risk of CAD. These candidates require annual testing, particularly if the program has a quick time to transplantation. If the transplant candidate has a history of diabetes, peripheral

---

Box 5
Criteria for cardiac stress testing at the time of referral

Prior history of cardiovascular disease

History of diabetes

History of smoking

Greater than 1 year on dialysis

Left ventricular hypertrophy

Hypertension

Hyperlipidemia

vascular disease, cardiovascular disease, cerebrovascular disease, or tobacco abuse, an annual imaging stress test should be required. If the transplant candidate is older than 60 years of age an annual imaging stress test should also be required.

Candidates who have suffered a recent cardiac event must provide all records from their cardiologist to be reviewed by the transplant center and the transplant cardiologist for appropriate assessment and testing. If testing is performed at a site not affiliated with the transplant program, is important to evaluate the test adequacy of the testing that was performed. Unless approved by the transplant center and the transplant cardiologist, all cardiac testing should be performed locally.

We recommend all programs develop criteria, in collaboration with a cardiologist, for acceptable modes of testing and establish their own acceptable limits. These can include exercise stress-echocardiogram. These are acceptable only for those patients able to achieve an adequate heart rate and rate-pressure product. In patients who are unable to perform adequately on a treadmill for any number of reasons, an adenosine-thallium or dobutamine stress echocardiogram ensures an adequate heart rate or rate-pressure product. Tests must be adequate to determine if cardiac ischemia is present at a high cardiac work load. The rate-pressure product achieved needs to be greater than 90% of the maximum and the achieved heart rate should also be greater than 90% of the predicted heart rate. If the test is inadequate, it is nondiagnostic. All submaximal stress tests should be repeated to avoid the possibility of missing an occult cardiac lesion. Because the objective behind cardiac testing is to avoid the possibility of a post-transplant myocardial infarction, any abnormal stress test suspicious for ischemia must be followed by a cardiac catheterization to determine if there is any large vessel cardiac disease that can be corrected.

Pulmonary hypertension (PHTN) is also commonly associated with chronic kidney disease and with increased mortality.[46] Patients with an estimated pulmonary artery systolic pressure of greater than 45 mm Hg by echocardiogram should undergo right heart catheterization for formal assessment. Factors associated with PHTN should be evaluated. If obvious factors, such as sleep apnea, thromboembolic pulmonary disease, or left heart failure, are not present, consultation with a pulmonologist to evaluate possible intrinsic lung disease should be pursued. If in fact, the transplant candidate is found to have PHTN characterized by a mean pulmonary artery pressure greater than 25 mm Hg, LVEDP (left ventricular end diastolic pressure) less than 15 mm Hg and pulmonary vascular resistance greater than 3 Woods units, the patient should be evaluated by a physician with expertise in the management of PHTN.

Patients on midodrine also require careful and insightful cardiac evaluation. Midodrine is an effective therapeutic option for the management of various forms of orthostatic hypotension (OH). Although there are many different etiologies for OH ranging from Parkinson disease to pure autonomic failure,[47] patients with diabetes on hemodialysis are prone to developing autonomic dysfunction that affects peripheral and central nervous system function. Neurogenic OH results from reduction of adrenergic nerve function. As such, some patients with diabetes are prone to developing postural hypotension between dialysis sessions. Although these patients have poorly functioning adrenergic input, their α-adrenergic receptors are intact and midodrine is commonly used to prevent symptomatic hypotension and decrease complications associated with hypotension during dialysis.

There are commonly two populations of patients with ESRD with OH who are supported with midodrine. One group requires support only during and immediately after dialysis and become orthostatic mainly because of volume losses. Another group is essentially on maintenance therapy to support their blood pressure. Although midodrine has been shown to be effective in small cohorts of transplant recipients,[48] requiring maintenance midodrine may be a poor prognostic sign and has been associated delayed graft function, graft failure, and death.[49] Therefore, candidates with history of OH who are on midodrine should be approached with a great deal of caution because they are at increased risk of poor outcomes and may be better left on maintenance dialysis.

PERIOPERATIVE SURGICAL ISSUES

The kidney transplant procedure starts with a right or left lower quadrant incision (**Fig. 1**A) to access the retroperitoneum to expose the common and/or external iliac artery and vein (**Fig. 1**B). Many of the risk factors that portend toward renal disease, specifically diabetes, hypertension, and smoking, also portend toward peripheral vascular disease. Moreover, renal dysfunction is associated with maladaptive calcium metabolism and vascular calcification.[43] As such, it is not surprising to find densely calcified arteries in transplant patients during the evaluation phase. When these prohibitive lesions are found early in the process, revascularization can be performed before a transplant[50] and may involve aortobiliac bypass, aortobifemoral bypass, or iliofemoral bypasses using prosthetic grafts. The transplant is subsequently performed safely onto the prosthesis through a standard retroperitoneal approach. Although most of these should be found during the preoperative evaluation, some are found at the time of the transplant procedure. Many surgeons have traditionally aborted the transplant when dense atherosclerosis is encountered. However, we, and others, have found this does not present an absolute need to abandon the transplant. Coosemans and coworkers[51] reports performing transplants in patients with vascular disease in three separate settings pretransplant, post-transplant, and simultaneously with six iliofemoral bypasses, one aortobiliac bypass, and one aortobifemoral bypass. All were performed with prosthetic grafts and the renal allograft was sewn into the side of the prosthetic.

Fortunately, most kidney transplants are performed with an end-to-side anastomosis directly to either the common or external iliac vein (**Fig. 2**A) and artery (**Fig. 2**B). We routinely perform the venous anastomosis first and place a bulldog clamp on the vein to allow us to test the integrity of the venous anastomosis. We find it is much easier to manage venous bleeding before fashioning the arterial anastomosis. We also administer furosemide and mannitol before completing the arterial anastomosis and reperfusing the kidney to mitigate reperfusion injury. Once we have ruled out any immediate risk of bleeding and are comfortable with the gross appearance of the kidney and reperfusion (**Fig. 3**A), we verify distal flow into the lower extremity by evaluating the iliac artery distal to the anastomosis and perform an intraoperative ultrasound to verify flow throughout the allograft.

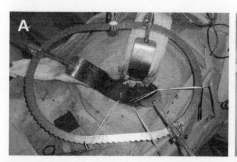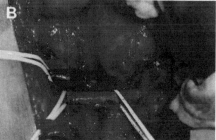

Fig. 1. Lower quadrant incision (*A*). Iliac artery and vein (*B*).

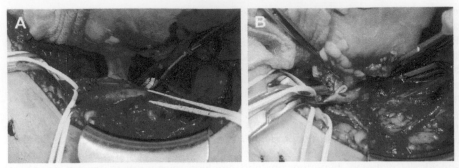

Fig. 2. End-to-side anastomosis, directly to the common or external iliac vein (A) and artery (B).

Once hemostasis is certain and the allograft is well perfused, we proceed with the ureteral anastomosis. The ureteroneocystostomy is performed in an end-to-side manner over a double J-stent. The benefits of using a stent include maintaining patency of ureter while the anastomosis is healing and reducing anatomic torsion. There are risks to using stents that include an increased risk of urinary tract infections (UTI), hematuria, stent migration, and an additional procedure for stent removal. Despite these potential risks, stents have been found to reduce the incidence of major urologic complications.[52] As such, our practice is to stent all transplanted ureters. Although UTIs seem to be more common, the occurrence is reduced with prophylactic antimicrobial agents. These agents, specifically sulfamethoxizole, are used to prevent opportunistic *Pneumocystis pneumonia* and provide the additional benefit of prophylaxis from UTI allowing us to use stents liberally. We routinely remove stents at 4 to 6 weeks to avoid encrustation and migration. All stents are removed by one of our consulting urologists in clinic with little consequence.

POSTOPERATIVE GRAFT DYSFUNCTION/ACUTE TUBULAR NECROSIS/DELAYED GRAFT FUNCTION

All renal allografts are at risk for postoperative acute tubular necrosis (ATN). ATN is associated with long cold and warm ischemic times, and cadaveric organs. At the time of reperfusion, most allografts make some urine (**Fig. 3**B). Urine output may fall

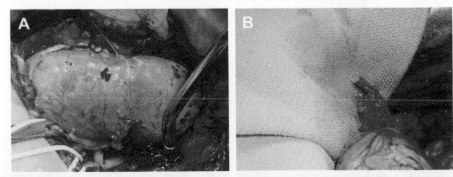

Fig. 3. Gross appearance of the kidney after reperfusion (A). Urine production after reperfusion (B).

to only milliliters an hour shortly after recovery. When a kidney has low or no urine output after recovery, an ultrasound is a critical component of the evaluation (**Fig. 4**). If ultrasound reveals good flow and there is no response to volume or diuretics, decrease IVF to avoid the evolution of pulmonary edema with congestive heart failure, and plan early dialysis (**Fig. 5**). The greatest likelihood is the graft dysfunction is secondary to ATN.

In general, the maximum fluid bolus should be 500 to 1000 mL. Overdoing fluid resuscitation in ATN only brings about pulmonary edema and the need for emergent dialysis. If blood flow is not found by ultrasound, the recipient should be taken back to the operating room for intraoperative assessment of blood flow. The quality of an ultrasound is affected by a patient's body habitus; as such, intraoperative evaluation is paramount to diagnose blood flow accurately. The only opportunity one has to intervene is early. As such, it should not be assumed the ultrasound is poor quality. Moreover, there are other causes of poor flow that have the capacity to compromise outcomes. Renal allograft compartment syndrome is characterized by increased pressure on the transplanted kidney in the iliac fossa that can lead to a reduction of the blood supply to the graft, resulting in organ ischemia.[53] Poor flow demonstrated by ultrasound may be the result of renal allograft compartment syndrome requiring surgical decompression of the graft and the subsequent placement of the kidney into the peritoneum by creating a peritoneal window or closing the incision in a tension-free manner.

If there are no unusual circumstances identified by the ultrasound and the recipient remains hemodynamically stable with no evidence of graft function by 5 to 7 days, a nuclear medicine scan is obtained to assess flow and function. If there is a suspicion of rejection, an ultrasound-guided biopsy is obtained no earlier than postoperative Day 7. If the biopsy is done earlier than Day 7, evolving rejection may be missed. If the biopsy reveals ATN, plans for discharge on dialysis can be made. If the biopsy reveals rejection, therapy depends on the type of rejection elucidated by the biopsy.

POSTOPERATIVE CARDIAC ISCHEMIA OR ARRHYTHMIA

The most common life-threatening complication following kidney transplant is life-threatening cardiac ischemia. Despite extensive preoperative screening and optimization, patients with ESRD are at high risk for postoperative myocardial events. An EKG

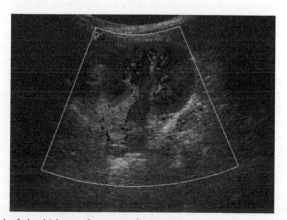

Fig. 4. Ultrasound of the kidney after reperfusion.

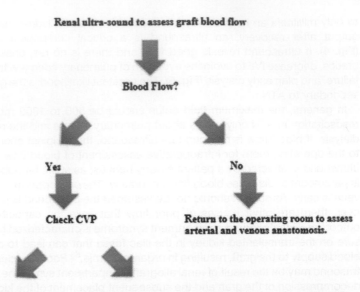

Fig. 5. Algorithm for low urine output. CVP, central venous pressure; IV, intravenous.

is obtained as part of the routine postoperative recovery. If there are any suspicious changes, serial troponins and EKGs are obtained every 8 hours for 24 hours. Although a single elevated troponin is not unusual because it is cleared by the kidney, a rising trend with EKG changes is concerning for a cardiac event. If a cardiac event is suspected, a cardiology consultation should be obtained, and an echocardiogram to evaluate the left ventricular function. Delayed graft function can sometimes be related to poor perfusion related to previously undiagnosed or new deterioration in cardiac performance.

VASCULAR COMPLICATIONS
Renal Artery Thrombosis

Renal artery thrombosis generally occurs early in the postoperatively period. This dreaded complication occurs infrequently with an incidence of less than 1%. This is a technical complication that can occur anywhere along a continuum starting with the organ recovery. Undo traction on the kidney during the recovery procedure can produce a tear in the renal artery intima and may go unrecognized during the back-table procedure. Interestingly, the back-table preparation and the implantation procedure can also be a source of intimal injury that leads to exposure of tissue factor and thrombosis or intimal dissection within the artery and subsequent thrombosis. Poor orientation can also produce torsion of donor renal artery that may culminate in thrombosis. When thrombosis is not the result of a technical misadventure, hypotension, multiple renal arteries, small donor arteries, and young donor age (<10 years of age) are risk factors for thrombosis. Finally, hyperacute rejection, refractory acute rejection, and hypercoagulable states also increase the risk of thrombosis.

The diagnosis has to be suspected to identify the event. This usually occurs when previously brisk urine output suddenly decreases. The diagnosis is confirmed by an emergent Doppler ultrasound of kidney. Alternatively, segmental arterial thrombosis may be asymptomatic or present with increasing creatinine, hypertension, or ureteric complication as a result of ischemia. If the diagnosis is made early in the course, the recipient is taken to the operating room for emergent exploration with arterial thrombectomy and anastomotic revision. When a revision is attempted, the allograft is explanted and flushed with heparin and preservative solution at 4°C. The kidney should flush well before an attempt is made to reperfuse. Unfortunately, most kidneys require removal, even when they flush well, because of prolonged warm ischemic time with dense thrombosis. Although there are reports of salvage of late thrombosis,[54] this is uncommon if not rare. Rouviere and co-workers[54] treated four patients with intra-arterial fibrinolysis for acute transplant artery thrombosis. Tissue plasminogen activator was used in one and urokinase in three. The patients presented with anuria for 13, 19, 20, and 48 hours. Two of the four allografts were salvaged with good function and each had been anuric for 19 and 20 hours before thrombolytics. Allograft nephrectomy secondary to thrombosis should not be viewed as a contraindication to a subsequent transplant.[55] Patients who suffer arterial occlusion secondary to thrombosis should undergo an extensive immunologic work-up to be certain the event was not the result of an immune-mediated event. Work-up includes classical HLA-mediated pathways and nonclassical activation of the immune system, such as antiplatelet or antiendothelial antibodies. Moreover, a hypercoagulable work-up before embarking on another transplant is critical and those found to have a thrombophilic disorder should receive perioperative anticoagulation.

Transplant Renal Artery Stenosis

The reported incidence of renal artery stenosis varies from 1% to 23% suggesting a lack of uncertainty with the true occurrence. The diagnosis is generally made beyond 3 to 6 months post-transplant. The most common site for stenosis is at the anastomosis and is seen with greater frequency with end-to-end anastomoses when the internal iliac is used to reperfuse the allograft. Although clinicians tend to recognize this at the level of the anastomosis and commonly occurs as a result of intimal hyperplasia, it can also be caused by recipient-related factors, such as iliac atherosclerotic disease, or from transplant-related factors including rejection, turbulent flow from a mal-positioned graft, or arterial misorientation and torsion. Patients who evolve renal artery stenosis may present with severe, refractory hypertension, and peripheral edema caused by activation of renin-angiotensin II-aldosterone axis. On examination, they may be found to have developed an audible bruit over the allograft, or they may be found to have a rising creatinine caused by allograft dysfunction. The diagnosis is made by a Doppler ultrasound demonstrating a greater than 20 mm Hg pressure difference across stenotic region, generally at the anastomosis.

The diagnosis is confirmed with an arteriogram. This is ideal because it can also be therapeutic. A nonoperative approach to transplant renal artery has emerged as the treatment of choice. Angioplasty with or without stent has excellent results.[56] When used alone, angioplasty has a 72% 1-year primary patency rate and an 85% 1-year secondary patency rate. When used in conjunction with a stent, angioplasty has a 100% primary patency rate at a mean of 18-month follow-up. Complications with angioplasty include arterial rupture, thrombosis, and graft loss. Operative revision of arterial stenosis should only be done for refractory stenosis, if at all. This is performed with nephrectomy, flushing, and reconstruction with vein patch angioplasty or autogenous venous bypass followed by reimplantation. It is critical to remember that these patients commonly present with increasing hypertension and new bruit over the allograft, with or without a rising creatinine. Because they still have a functioning allograft, there is questionable benefit to an attempted revision given substantial morbidities and mortality. Operative revision is associated with a perioperative graft loss rate of 5% to 10%, ureteral injury of 10% to 15%, and mortality of 5%.

RECIPIENT ARTERIAL COMPLICATIONS
Iliac Artery Thrombosis

Iliac artery injuries with thrombosis commonly occur as a result of clamp injuries. The diagnosis is made on physical examination when an ischemic extremity is identified during the early post-transplant period. Late diagnosis of this feared complication is often avoided by a routine intraoperative examination of the iliac artery distal to the anastomosis. When the diagnosis is not obvious intraoperatively, diligent vascular examination of both extremities before and after surgery is suggestive of malperfusion. A duplex examination or angiogram confirms the diagnosis. These patients should be managed operatively with balloon thrombectomy and patch angioplasty.

Iliac Artery Stenosis

Iliac arterial stenosis presents more chronically than thrombosis. Patients may present with allograft dysfunction, or hypertension mimicking renal arterial stenosis clinically. They may also present with classic signs of peripheral vascular disease, such as gluteal claudication with or without diminished femoral pulses. Iliac artery stenosis is commonly the result of progressive peripheral vascular disease and management includes angioplasty with stenting and is very successful.

RENAL VEIN THROMBOSIS

Renal vein thrombosis occurs early within the first 10 days post-transplant. The reported incidence is on the order of 0.5% to 3.4% and is associated with multiple etiologies. The vein is pliable and vulnerable to angulation and torsion affecting flow. It is particularly subject to these flow-limiting influences when the renal vein has an excessive length. A narrowed outflow tract at the anastomosis related to overly tight suturing technique also limits flow. These turbulent flow dynamics, in the extreme, end in thrombosis within the renal vein. Because the vein is pliable, it is also affected by external forces and can easily be compressed by a hematoma or lymphocele. Another possible mechanism that results in renal vein thrombosis involves an extension of an iliac vein thrombosis. These may be associated with hypercoagulable states.

Patients may have a variety of symptoms including a precipitous decrease in urine output with a tender swollen graft. They may also have hematuria or may be completely asymptomatic and present with rising creatinine. Alternatively, they may complain of lower extremity edema or pain. The diagnosis of renal vein thrombosis is commonly made with a Doppler ultrasound demonstrating a lack of flow in renal vein, and reversal of diastolic arterial flow. Occasionally, the diagnosis is made after an initial diagnosis of femoral or iliac vein thrombosis. Once diagnosed, renal vein thrombosis is an operative emergency mandating exploration to avoid graft rupture. Thrombectomy can be attempted when the diagnosis is made virtually immediately but most patients require allograft nephrectomy.

RECIPIENT VENOUS COMPLICATIONS

Iliofemoral thromboembolism most commonly occurs in the early period following a transplant. When this occurs early after surgery, it usually occurs in association with operative factors. When it occurs late, it is seen beyond 4 weeks after the transplant and may be associated with increasing hematocrit with robust production or erythropoietin. Risk factors include recipient age (>40), diabetes, known hypercoagulable states, and prior history of deep venous thrombosis. Iliofemoral thrombosis has a reported incidence of 5% deep venous thrombosis rate, and 1% pulmonary embolism. High-risk patients should receive perioperative low-dose heparin prophylactically.

RENAL ALLOGRAFT ARTERIOVENOUS FISTULA

Allograft arteriovenous fistula occur following percutaneous allograft biopsy. This complication occurs most commonly when the biopsy is performed of medullary rather than cortical regions. The diagnosis is made by Doppler ultrasound revealing abnormally high-velocities with turbulent flow isolated to a single segmental or interlobar artery and paired vein. Arteriovenous fistulae are usually small, asymptomatic, and resolve spontaneously. When they are large or enlarging, selective segmental arterial embolization is the preferred intervention with steel coils used as embolization material.

ANEURYSMS

These are rare entities but when aneurysms occur, they arise from anastomotic disruption of the renal artery. The most common cause is infection in an immunosuppressed setting. The diagnosis is often incidental on Doppler ultrasound for nonspecific causes. If the patient is stable, the ultrasound findings are confirmed with an arteriogram. There is an enormous risk of free rupture and pathognomonic signs include symptoms of local pressure that will certainly be followed by hypotensive shock. These patients should be taken immediately to the operating room for allograft nephrectomy. Attempts to repair are futile and one should concentrate on saving the patient over the graft.

BLEEDING AFTER TRANSPLANT

Patients undergoing a renal transplant have, at baseline, a platelet dysfunction related to uremia. Although gross bleeding is uncommon, it is not unusual to need to exert some effort establishing hemostasis as the raw surfaces of the retroperitoneum ooze related to the underlying uremic platelets. More significant bleeding usually originates from a suboptimal back-table preparation and unidentified vessels in graft hilum may bleed. This is avoided with a careful back-table preparation of allograft. Specifically, excessive dissection of renal hilum is not recommended. Another source is bleeding from retroperitoneal vessels. These vessels undergo vasospasm intraoperatively and start bleeding postoperatively when perfusion to kidney improves and are at greater risk of bleeding as the patient becomes progressively more hypertensive postoperatively. This is prevented by a careful methodical search for bleeders and evaluation of the retroperitoneum at the end of the transplant.

Massive postoperative hemorrhage after an unremarkable anastomosis may indicate venous anastomotic disruption.[57] This is not uncommon when patients awake violently from anesthesia with forceful Valsalva tearing the venous anastomosis. Risk factors for venous disruption include short right renal vein[58] in an obese recipient, and obesity itself. Another source of significant postoperative hemorrhage includes preoperative antiplatelet therapy, anticoagulation, or postoperative heparinization. Signs and symptoms of serious bleeding include tachycardia and associated hypotension, decreasing urine output, decreasing central venous pressure, and increasing flank or lower quadrant pain with distention. The diagnosis should be suspected and efforts to diagnose and treat should not be delayed. One can either elect to go straight to the operating room when the clinical suspicion is high or an ultrasound, or obtain a noncontrast computed tomography scan to assist in making the diagnosis.

Management may include observation if the recipient is hemodynamically stable and graft function is not affected. If the bleeding is from a venous source, it usually stops spontaneously. A desire to correct uremic platelet dysfunction with desmopressin or estrogen should be avoided because this may lead to allograft thrombosis. Similarly, other hemostatic drugs, such as factor VIIa, should be avoided for similar fears. If the patient is hemodynamically unstable, requiring ongoing transfusions, or if graft function is at risk because of hypovolemia or compression, surgical exploration should be pursued. Operative management involves evacuation of the forming hematoma, and search for culprit bleeder, which is often not found.

HEMATOMA

Patients with uremia have a predisposition for bleeding as a result of platelet dysfunction. These patients are at higher than usual risk for postoperative wound and perigraft hematoma formation. Hematomas tend to develop slowly and present late during the postoperative recovery. If a transplant recipient develops a hematoma, they may complain of pain and tenderness. Significant hematomas can require operative evacuation to avoid venous and ureteral compression. An unexplained drop in hematocrit must be investigated. First, obtain an ultrasound to evaluate the retroperitoneal kidney for evidence of fluid around the kidney that may represent blood. If there is evidence of venous outflow obstruction or significant hydronephrosis with a large perigraft fluid collection, the suspected hematoma should be evacuated because it may result in dysfunction or compromise the renal allograft. If the patient is large, limiting the effectiveness of the ultrasound, a noncontrast computed tomography should be obtained to rule out a significant fluid accumulation suggestive of hematoma.

BLEEDING AFTER PERCUTANEOUS BIOPSY

One of the downsides of protocol biopsies is bleeding. The reported incidence of bleeding after a biopsy is 8%.[59] Bleeding may be prevented by targeting the renal cortex and avoiding medullary tissue. Patients should undergo frequent vital sign monitoring after a percutaneous biopsy, and remain at bedrest with pressure over the biopsy site for 6 hours. At the completion of the period of bedrest, a hematocrit should be checked to rule out occult, asymptomatic, bleeding. Bleeding after a biopsy commonly tamponades. As such, observation with serial vitals and hematocrits usually is sufficient. However, surgical exploration is generally necessary for clinical instability or ongoing transfusion requirement. Percutaneous superselective segmental renal artery embolization has been successful with no harmful effects on the allograft function in six patients.[60]

BLEEDING AFTER TRANSPLANT NEPHRECTOMY

If the allograft nephrectomy was performed because of local infection at transplant site, consideration should be given to ligation of iliac artery with extra-anatomic bypass because of an increased risk of stump blow out from residual infection following mycotic aneurysm formation with rupture.[61]

UROLOGIC COMPLICATIONS

Although urologic complications are not uncommon, graft loss is rarely the result of a urologic complication. Urologic complications range from UTIs that are seen in up to 80% of cases to urinary leaks that occur in 3% to 10% of the time. Ureteral obstruction and stenosis are observed in approximately 2% to 15% of all transplants and vesicoureteral reflux is difficult to quantify because it is seen with some frequency but is rarely of consequence.

Urinary Tract Infections

UTIs are the most common urologic complication encountered affecting nearly half of kidney transplant recipients in the first year after transplantation. The most common organisms cultured are *Enterococcus faecalis* and *Escherichia coli*. Females tend to be at greater risk for infection, and immunosuppression and the presence of a double-J ureteral stent significantly increases the risk. Most patients have asymptomatic bacteriuria likely as a result of being on prophylaxis for *P pneumonia* and a smaller percentage develop symptomatic UTIs. UTIs can induce substantial morbidity in immunosuppressed patients with risk of pyelonephritis and urosepsis. Treatment of asymptomatic bacteriuria may be beneficial to prevent subsequent episodes of symptomatic UTIs.[62]

Urine Leaks

Urine leaks do not occur with any great frequency.[63] Patients develop pain and swelling at transplant site usually within 1 week of the transplant. Although perinephric fluid can be aspirated and evaluated for creatinine, a mercapto-acetyl-triglycine scan or nuclear medicine renal scan is the most sensitive diagnostic test to establish the presence of a urine leak.[64] A urine leak can occur anywhere along the urinary tract, but the most common site of a leak is at the distal end. The distal ureter is commonly at risk because of ischemia from devascularization during the recovery and/or back-table preparation. A leak can also occur at the ureteroneocystostomy as a result of technical complications. The proximal ureter is rarely the site of a urine leak. Management varies depending on the degree of leak. A small leak can usually be managed with prolonged Foley drainage to allow healing of the defect. A more significant leak may occasionally be amenable to management with a percutaneous stent but generally requires reoperation, sometimes at the expense of the kidney. Occasionally, complete ureteral necrosis can occur as a result of an organ recovery injury. Ureteral injury can also occur secondary to compression by a hematoma or as a manifestation of rejection. This requires reoperation with ureteral reconstruction using one of two techniques: a complicated bladder reconstruction with a psoas hitch or Boari flap or revision with a ureteroureterostomy using the recipient's native ipsilateral or contralateral ureter.

Ureteral Obstruction/Stenosis

Ureteral obstructions can occur early or late in the course of a transplant and can have multiple etiologies. When an obstruction occurs early, it is usually the result of technical error, edema, hematoma, presence of unknown donor nephrolithiasis, perirenal fluid collection (hematoma, urinoma, abscess, lymphocele), or bladder dysfunction. When a ureteral obstruction occurs well after a transplant, it may be the result of periureteral fibrosis, formation of nephrolithiasis, chronic ischemia of the distal ureter resulting in stricture, primary uroepithelial malignancy, PTLD, or BK virus–nephropathy secondary to polyoma virus. However, the most common cause of ureteral stenosis is ischemia. Because the blood supply to the transplanted ureter is derived primarily from the hilar renal vessels, stenosis usually occurs in the distal ureter. When these strictures occur early in the post-transplant course, it is usually the result of a technical complication, ureteral skeletonization, associated with the organ recovery or the back-table preparation.

Ultrasound is one of the staples for evaluation of a renal transplant recipient in the early postoperative course and at any time following a transplant as part of the evaluation of a change in creatinine or localized allograft discomfort. The diagnosis of ureteral stricture is initially established by an allograft ultrasound demonstrating significant hydronephrosis. The initial treatment of a ureteral stricture involves consultation with interventional radiology and placement of a nephrostomy tube. Once the renal function normalizes, a ureterogram (**Fig. 6**) establishes the location and length of the stricture. Noninvasive approaches to short strictures include balloon dilation, or laser incision with stenting. If the stricture is long or attempts to open a short stricture fail, then operative approaches include ureteroureterostomy using the ipsilateral or contralateral native ureter. During the course of mobilizing the native ureter, it is critical not to devascularize the ureter. As such, mobilization should be left to a minimum. The donor ureter is freshened back to a viable, well-vascularized segment of ureter and the repair is done in an end-to-side or end-to-end fashion. If there is sufficient length in the donor ureter, reimplantation of the donor ureter with redo ureteroneocystostomy is a viable option. In rare instances, when there is no native ureter, and when a reimplantation is not an option, a Boari flap is a viable option.

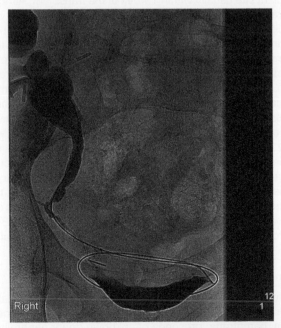

Fig. 6. Algorithm for low urine output starts with obtaining an ultrasound to evaluate blood flow. If good blood in-flow is visualized without venous outflow obstruction and no evidence of massive hydronephrosis, then check a central venous pressure (CVP). If the CVP is less than 10 mm Hg, administer fluid bolus. If the CVP is greater than 10 mm Hg, administer Lasix and diuril. If the ultrasound does not demonstrate adequate blood flow or reveals massive hydronephrosis, return to the operating room (OR) for direct inspection.

Urinary Retention

Male transplant recipients are at risk for developing postoperative urinary retention following a kidney transplant.[65] Benign prostatic hypertrophy is underappreciated in anuric patients with ESRD, and failure of diagnosis in this population can lead to complications after kidney transplantation.[66] Urinary retention is also observed more commonly in patients with diabetes. Urinary retention is, theoretically, a risk for ureteral anastomotic disruption and for UTIs. Initial post-transplant treatment requires intermittent bladder catheterization and discharge with indwelling Foley catheter. Urinary tract complications are more common in these patients with benign prostatic hypertrophy. However, if the diagnosis of benign prostatic hypertrophy is made before transplant, being on medical therapy before transplantation reduces the incidence of these complications.[66] Patients with neurogenic bladders are also at risk for urinary retention. These patients are commonly treated with an ileal conduit or augmentation cystoplasty well before transplant,[67] and the donor ureter is sewn to the augmentation or ileal conduit.

Hematuria

Post-transplant hematuria has a bimodal distribution. It is seen early post-transplant and is usually associated with bleeding at the ureteral anastomosis. Rarely, the hematuria is significant turning the urine into a dark cabernet color with obvious clots. When this occurs, patients develop urethral outflow obstruction with bladder distention. Decompression is critical with a large, three-way hematuria catheter connected to continuous irrigation. The irrigation should not be connected to a pressure pump but should be allowed to flow freely with gravity and should be titrated to the color of the output. As the urine becomes a lighter color, the rate of flow is reduced until the hematuria resolves. These early, anastomotic bleeds rarely require an operative intervention. When the hematuria occurs later in the post-transplant course, the causes are varied and range from benign to malignant etiologies (**Box 6**) involving both the native and transplanted kidney and may require biopsy of the allograft or formal urologic evaluation including cystoscopy.[68]

LYMPHOCELE

The retroperitoneal dissection to prepare for a transplant involves skeletonization of the iliac artery and vein. As such, an extensive network of lymphatics that drain the lower extremities are divided. It is not uncommon to develop a lymphocele from lymph leaking out of these lymphatic channels. Lymphoceles have the capacity of growing to

---

Box 6
Causes of late hematuria

Urolithiasis

Benign bladder mucosal bleeding

Bladder cancer

Uroepithelial malignancy of the ureter

Kidney cancer from the native kidney

Kidney cancer from the transplanted kidney

Histologic allograft pathology requiring biopsy: chronic rejection, IgA nephropathy, cyclosporine toxicity, acute rejection, focal segmental glomerulosclerosis, glomerulonephritis, tubular atrophy, and interstitial fibrosis

sufficient volumes that can compress either the ureter or vein producing allograft dysfunction commonly characterized by a rising creatinine. The diagnosis is routinely made with an ultrasound. If the graft function has been affected, the first step in management includes drainage. Once the fluid is demonstrated to be a lymphocele, sclerotherapy is effective after optimal drainage has been attained. In circumstances when sclerotherapy is not effective, a peritoneal window created laparoscopically or though laparotomy effectively resolves all lymphoceles.

REJECTION

Hyperacute/humoral rejection is a rare event in the current era of transplantation. This was seen historically before the modern era of solid-phase antibody detection and characterization. Hyperacute rejection is mediated by preformed donor-specific antibodies (DSA) that are produced after exposure to antigens. This exposure is usually in the form of a sensitizing event that occurs with blood transfusions, pregnancy with an Rh disparate pregnancy, or prior transplant. We do not see this type of rejection with any frequency because our ability to characterize these antibodies allows us to avoid donors known to have the antigens the antibodies would react against. Finally, the reliability of the crossmatch before the transplant definitively prevents using a kidney that would be the target of these DSA.

The incidence of acute rejection varies considerably and occurs somewhere between 10% and 50% within the first 6 months depending on a variety of immunologic variables including recipient DSA burden, donor/recipient match, degree of immunosuppression, allograft quality, and recipient and donor age. Acute rejection is seen in the first week post-transplant and is most common in the first 3 months. Acute rejection can result from cell-mediated immunity or antibody-mediated immunity. Occasionally, both processes are involved. Rejection occurs more frequently in patients that are heavily sensitized and those who experience early graft dysfunction associated with ATN. Early postoperative rejection responds, in most patients, to bolus steroids in the form of Solu-Medrol. Although dosing protocols vary from program to program, a conventional dosing includes 500 mg intravenous daily for 3 to 5 days. If patients do not respond and rejection is persistent on a repeat biopsy or there is aggressive rejection on the initial biopsy, thymoglobulin therapy is preferred.

Despite a negative cellular crossmatch, some patients experience humoral/antibody-mediated rejection. The diagnosis was classically made with special stains for C4-d deposition in the basement membrane of the glomerulus. Since the evolution of solid-state technology, we also make the diagnosis of humoral rejection by the detection of DSA in the proper clinical and histologic context. The cornerstone of therapy is to decrease the alloantibody titer. This is accomplished by plasmapheresis for 5 days or until a clinical response is observed. An antibody titer should be checked following plasmapheresis. If the titer remains high, a second or rarely third round of plasmapheresis should be performed. Plasmapheresis is followed by intravenous immunoglobulin (2 g/kg/dose). The treatment of antibody-mediated rejection has evolved considerably and programs use a variety of protocols involving plasmapheresis, intravenous immunoglobulin, in combination with varying doses of rituximab. Rituximab is an anti-CD20 antibody and causes cell death by binding the CD-20 receptor on B cells and has become an accepted adjunct in the treatment of humoral rejection. There are emerging reports of groups using bortezomib to treat antibody-mediated rejection refractory to conventional treatment, such as plasmapheresis, intravenous immunoglobulin, and rituximab.

HEMOLYTIC UREMIC SYNDROME

Although hemolytic uremic syndrome (HUS) is best described in the setting of *E coli*–associated infections in the general population, it is observed in the kidney transplant patient population in association with the use of immunosuppression. Also known as thrombotic microangiopathy, HUS is a well-described complication of calcineurin inhibitor use (cyclosporin or tacrolimus). It is believed to result from direct vascular injury. Calcineurin inhibitors may produce a direct toxic effect on vascular endothelium by interfering with the generation of endothelial prostacyclin. In patients whose renal failure was the result of HUS, it is difficult to distinguish between the two processes. However, the intimal changes or onion-skin lesions of interlobar arteries seen in HUS are not regular features of calcineurin inhibitor toxicity. Calcineurin inhibitor toxicity usually results in the deposition of bland thrombi within the lumen of arterioles and glomerular capillaries. Unlike true HUS, these lesions are not widespread or associated with extensive tissue necrosis.

Clinically, HUS presents with worsening renal function if in fact there was an initial improvement in function, hematuria, thrombocytopenia, microangiopathic hemolytic anemia on a blood smear, elevated lactate dehydrogenase, and depressed haptoglobin. Calcineurin inhibitor–induced HUS may not be readily apparent initially and the laboratory findings may not be consistent. Because this is an idiosyncratic reaction, calcineurin inhibitor levels may not be elevated to toxic levels. However, one must have an index of suspicion by either an initial drop in the patient's platelet count with an associated anemia and a rise in a previously falling creatinine to make the diagnosis. Once the diagnosis is contemplated, a biopsy needs to be performed. If the diagnosis is made, one can expect an improvement in function by changing the calcineurin inhibitor and instituting plasmapheresis.

Cytomegalovirus/Epstein-BARR VIRUS/POLYOMA VIRUS

CMV is not pathologic in an immune-competent host. There are well established risk factors for CMV infections. Once a person is infected with CMV (primary infection), the virus becomes latent in white blood cells. As such, donors, cadaveric and living, who have been previously infected with CMV are able to transmit CMV infection to immunosuppressed solid organ transplant (SOT) recipients.

Donor-to-recipient mismatch is the most common and well-identified risk factor for developing a CMV infection. Allograft rejection is another well-established risk factor because treatment of rejection usually weakens the immune system further, which serves to increase the susceptibility to CMV infection. Kidney transplant recipients may develop CMV infections post-transplant involving virtually any and all organ systems with varied presentations. CMV syndrome is the most common presentation with fever, and any number of constitutional symptoms including generalized malaise, leukopenia, lymphocytosis, thrombocytopenia, pancreatitis, and elevated hepatic enzymes with detectable copies of CMV in the serum by quantitative assay. Tissue-invasive CMV disease is different from CMV syndrome in that there must be evidence of CMV on biopsy of the specific organ or tissue (CMV in cerebrospinal fluid for central nervous system disease). Patients manifest signs and symptoms associated with the organ system involved, such as encephalitis and retinitis, hepatitis, colitis, and pneumonitis. It is important to recognize that although all organ systems are susceptible to tissue-invasive disease, the transplanted organ is most susceptible. Therefore, renal dysfunction is a manifestation of tissue invasiveness in kidney transplant recipients. As such, a biopsy is critical to establish an unresolved source of a rising creatinine before deciding on a course of treatment. For instance, we believe it is imprudent to pulse a given patient with steroids on a whim that their rising creatinine is caused by rejection because it could be caused by infection. The steroid pulse would only aggravate, if not prevent, the recovery. As such, a biopsy is critical to be certain of the most appropriate course of action. Ironically, symptomatic CMV infection or CMV disease has been identified as a factor that increases the risk for subsequent rejection in kidney transplant recipients.[69]

Although the ideal circumstance is to match donor and recipient CMV status, it is impractical because the organ supply already limits the ability to transplant more liberally. Although our recommendation is that high-risk, CMV-mismatched (CMV-negative recipients of CMV-positive donor kidneys) recipients and patients treated with thymoglobulin (whether as induction or for rejection) should receive universal prophylaxis, there are other strategies. Programs must decide what approach makes greatest sense in their programmatic philosophy. One strategy involves prophylaxis against CMV with antiviral agents. In this strategy, all SOT recipients receive therapy during the highest period of immunosuppression, the period of greatest risk. The issue that programs need to sort out is the cost associated with treating everyone, and the risk of inducing resistance by treating everyone. Another strategy involves preemptive treatment that is administered based on detection of asymptomatic viral replication in blood. This strategy requires serial monitoring with a quantitative detection assay.

EBV has been found to induce a type of lymphoma in recipients of SOT known as PTLD.[39] EBV-infected B cells undergo clonal transformation in the immunosuppressed recipient producing PTLD, which has also been found to develop in T-cell clones. Risk factors for developing PTLD include primary EBV infection in a seronegative recipient of a seropositive donor organ, particularly, in the setting of strong immunosuppression with thymoglobulin or stronger agents. An associated history of CMV coinfection has also been shown to be a risk factor for developing PTLD. Clinical manifestation ranges from febrile mononucleosis-like illness with lymphadenopathy to the formation of solid, extranodal masses. Central nervous system involvement is not uncommon and involvement of the transplanted allograft is seen frequently.

The diagnosis of PTLD requires a tissue biopsy and the subsequent classification is based on histologic findings and clonal expansion. Although withdrawal or reduction of immunosuppression is widely accepted as the first-line strategy for the treatment of PTLD, the role of additional therapeutic interventions has evolved.[70] Rituximab, an anti-CD20 monoclonal antibody, has proven effective in treatment of EBV-driven PTLD.[71]

Polyomavirus (BKV) is a ubiquitous, DNA virus with the primary infection occurring in the urinary tract during childhood. Most of the worldwide population (80%) are seropositive for BKV. Following resolution of the primary infection, the virus lies dormant in the renal and uroepithelial cells. BKV may cause nephropathy in the allograft of an immunosuppressed transplant recipient. BKV nephropathy has an incidence of approximately 15% with most cases occurring within 1 year of the transplant. The manifestation is an unexplained renal dysfunction. The greatest risk factor for reactivation from latency is immunosuppression. Patients who have been treated for prior rejection seem to have an increased risk, as do older recipients and male recipients of cadaveric allografts.[72]

Early diagnosis is critical to averting BKV–associated nephropathy (BKAN) and its sequelae. As such, our recommendation is to perform quantitative assay every 3 months for the first 2 years with a need to reduce immunotherapy at the initial detection of any viral copies. If any degree of allograft dysfunction is noted, a biopsy needs to be performed because a definitive diagnosis of BKAN requires allograft biopsy.[73] It is important to distinguish BKAN from rejection because the treatments are diametrically opposed. Serum polymerase chain reaction is sensitive (100%) but less specific (88%).[74] Because the serum assay cannot rule out rejection, it is best used as indication for biopsy and to monitor response to therapy. As such, renal histopathology with immunohistochemistry or in situ hybridization is the gold standard for BKAN. Reduction in immunosuppression should be instituted before there is evidence of graft injury. Unfortunately, this strategy is not universally effective. To date, there have been several reports using either cidofovir or leflunomide with varying success.[75] Although the results have been modest, the side effects are significant. Finally, there are some groups that have reported success in treatment of BKAN with ciprofloxacin.[76]

SUMMARY

The incidence of ESRD has increased steadily over the last several decades. There has also been dramatic improvements in the outcomes following transplantation with a significant increase in the number of patients receiving renal-replacement therapy in the form of a transplant. This is caused by advances in surgical technique, improvements in immunosuppression, and better control of associated comorbid conditions.

Transplantation is transformative and offers the greatest potential for restoring a healthy, productive, and durable life to appropriately selected patients. Moreover, in an era when cost effectiveness is also being weighed into the equation of health care, transplantation offers the greatest good. It offers the best for patients who are appropriate candidates with the best resource use for the health care system. The key is in appropriate selection of candidates and the development of programs that foster behavioral modification that assist kidney transplant recipients maximize "the greatest good."

REFERENCES

1. Levey AS, Coresh J, Greene T, et al, Chronic Kidney Disease Epidemiology Collaboration. Using standardized serum creatinine values in the modification of diet in renal disease study equation for estimating glomerular filtration rate. Ann Intern Med 2006;145(4):247–54.
2. Levey AS, Stevens LA, Schmid CH, et al. A new equation to estimate glomerular filtration rate. Ann Intern Med 2009;150(9):604–12.
3. Washington (DC): National Academies Press (US); 1991. p. 176–205.
4. Wolfe RA, Ashby VB, Milford EL, et al. Comparison of mortality in all patients on dialysis, patients on dialysis awaiting transplantation, and recipients of a first cadaveric transplant. N Engl J Med 1999;341(23):1725–30.
5. United Network for Organ Sharing. Available at: https://unos.org/data/transplant-trendsbyorgan. Accessed June 1, 2018.
6. Kasiske BL, Cangro CB, Hariharan S, et al. The evaluation of renal transplant candidates: clinical practice guidelines. Am J Transplant 2001;2(Suppl. 1):5–95.
7. Rao PS, Merion RM, Ashby VB, et al. Kayler renal transplantation in elderly patients older than 70 years of age: results from the scientific registry of transplant recipients. Transplantation 2007;83(8):1069–74.
8. Giral M, Bertola JP, Foucher Y, et al. Effect of brain-dead donor resuscitation on delayed graft function: results of a monocentric analysis. Transplantation 2007;83:1174–81.
9. Guralnik JM, Simonsick EM, Ferrucci L, et al. A short physical performance battery assessing lower extremity function: association with self-reported disability

and prediction of mortality and nursing home admission. J Gerontol 1994;49(2): M85–94.

10. Fairhall N, Sherrington C, Cameron ID, et al. A multifactorial intervention for frail older people is more than twice as effective among those who are compliant: complier average causal effect analysis of a randomised trial. J Physiother 2017;63(1):40–4.

11. Freiberger E, de Vreede P, Schoene D, et al. Performance-based physical function in older community-dwelling persons: a systematic review of instruments. Age Ageing 2012;41(6):712–21.

12. Pavasini R, Guralnik J, Brown JC, et al. Short Physical Performance Battery and all-cause mortality: systematic review and meta-analysis. BMC Med 2016;14:215.

13. Fried LP, Tangen CM, Walston J, et al, Cardiovascular Health Study Collaborative Research Group. Frailty in older adults: evidence for a phenotype. J Gerontol A Biol Sci Med Sci 2001;56(3):M146–56.

14. McAdams-DeMarco MA, Law A, Salter ML, et al. Frailty as a novel predictor of mortality and hospitalization in individuals of all ages undergoing hemodialysis. J Am Geriatr Soc 2013;61(6):896–901.

15. McAdams-DeMarco MA, Law A, King E, et al. Frailty and mortality in kidney transplant recipients. Am J Transplant 2015;15(1):149–54.

16. de Roij van Zuijdewijn CL, ter Wee PM, Chapdelaine I, et al. A Comparison of 8 nutrition-related tests to predict mortality in hemodialysis patients. J Ren Nutr 2015;25(5):412–9.

17. Hanish SI, Petersen RP, Collins BH, et al. Obesity predicts increased overall complications following pancreas transplantation. Transplant Proc 2005;37(8): 3564–6.

18. Sood A, Hakim DN, Hakim NS. Consequences of recipient obesity on postoperative outcomes in a renal transplant: a systematic review and meta-analysis. Exp Clin Transplant 2016;14(2):121–8.

19. Maisonneuve P, Agodoa L, Gellert R, et al. Cancer in patients on dialysis for end-stage renal disease: an international collaborative study. Lancet 1999;354:93–9.

20. American Cancer Society Screening Guidelines. Available at: https://www.cancer.org/healthy/find-cancer-early/cancer-screening-guidelines. Accessed June 1, 2018.

21. Penn I. Evaluation of transplant candidates with pre-existing malignancies. Ann Transplant 1997;2:14–7.

22. Baddley JW, Winthrop KL, Patkar NM, et al. Curtis geographic distribution of endemic fungal infections among older persons, United States. Emerg Infect Dis 2011;17(9):1664–9. Available at: www.cdc.gov/eid.

23. Ekrikpo UE, Kengne AP, Bello AK, et al. Chronic kidney disease in the global adult HIV- infected population: a systematic review and meta-analysis. PLoS One 2018; 13(4):e0195443.

24. Marcus R, Favero MS, Banerjee S, et al. Prevalence and incidence of human immunodeficiency virus among patients undergoing long-term hemodialysis. The Cooperative Dialysis Study Group. Am J Med 1991;90:614–9.

25. Malat GE, Boyle SM, Jindal RM, et al. Kidney transplantation in HIV-positive patients: a single-center, 16-year experience. Am J Kidney Dis 2018 [pii:S0272-6386(18)30546-8]. [Epub ahead of print].

26. Ahuja TS, Zingman B, Glicklich D. Long-term survival in an HIV-infected renal transplant recipient. Am J Nephrol 1997;17:480–2.

27. Hussein MM, Mooij JM, Roujouleh H. Tuberculosis and chronic renal disease. Semin Dial 2003;16(1):38–44.

28. Segall L, Covic A. Diagnosis of tuberculosis in dialysis patients: current strategy. Clin J Am Soc Nephrol 2010;5(6):1114–22.
29. Costa SD, de Sandes-Freitas TV, Jacinto CN, et al. Tuberculosis after kidney transplantation is associated with significantly impaired allograft function. Transpl Infect Dis 2017;19(5). https://doi.org/10.1111/tid.12750.
30. Seyhan EC, Sökücü S, Altin S, et al. Comparison of the QuantiFERON-TB Gold In-Tube test with the tuberculin skin test for detecting latent tuberculosis infection in hemodialysis patients. Transpl Infect Dis 2010;12(2):98–105.
31. Goodkin DA, Bieber B, Jadoul M, et al. Mortality, hospitalization, and quality of life among patients with hepatitis C infection on hemodialysis. Clin J Am Soc Nephrol 2017;12(2):287–97.
32. Gane E, Pilmore H. Management of chronic viral hepatitis before and after renal transplantation. Transplantation 2002;74(4):427–37.
33. La Manna G. HCV and kidney transplant in the era of new direct-acting antiviral agents (DAAs). J Nephrol 2018;31(2):185–7.
34. Colombo M, Aghemo A, Liu H, et al. Treatment with ledipasvir-sofosbuvir for 12 or 24 weeks in kidney transplant recipients with chronic hepatitis C virus genotype 1 or 4 infection: a randomized trial. Ann Intern Med 2017;166(2):109–17.
35. Marinaki S, Kolovou K, Sakellariou S, et al. Hepatitis B in renal transplant patients. World J Hepatol 2017;9(25):1054–63.
36. Hsu C, Tsou HH, Lin SJ, et al. Chemotherapy-induced hepatitis B reactivation in lymphoma patients with resolved HBV infection: a prospective study. Hepatology 2014;59(6):2092–100.
37. Miao B, Lao XM, Lin GL. Post-transplant withdrawal of lamivudine results in fatal hepatitis flares in kidney transplant recipients, under immunosuppression, with inactive hepatitis B infection. Afr Health Sci 2016;16(4):1094–100.
38. Amon W, Farrell PJ. Reactivation of Epstein-Barr virus from latency. Rev Med Virol 2004;15(3):149–56.
39. Dharnidhrka VR, Webster AC, Martinez OM, et al. Post-transplant lymphoproliferative disorders. Nat Rev Dis Primers 2016;2:15088.
40. Danziger-Isakova L, Kumar D, the AST Infectious Diseases Community of Practice. Vaccination in solid organ transplantation. Am J Transplant 2013;13(Suppl 4):311–7.
41. Weinrauch LA, Claggett B, Liu J, et al. Smoking and outcomes in kidney transplant recipients: a post hoc survival analysis of the FAVORIT trial. Int J Nephrol Renovasc Dis 2018;11:155–64.
42. Aref A, Sharma A, Halawa A. Smoking in renal transplantation; facts beyond myth. World J Transplant 2017;7(2):129–33.
43. Henaut L, Chillon JM, Kamel S, et al. Updates on the mechanisms and the care of cardiovascular calcification in chronic kidney disease. Semin Nephrol 2018;38(3):233–50.
44. Di Lullo L, House A, Gorini A, et al. Chronic kidney disease and cardiovascular complications. Heart Fail Rev 2015;20(3):259–72.
45. Bilancio G, Celano M, Cozza V, et al. Early prediction of cardiovascular disease in kidney transplant recipients. Transplant Proc 2017;49(9):2092–8.
46. Thenappan T. Pulmonary hypertension in chronic kidney disease: a hemodynamic characterization. Pulm Circ 2017;7(3):567–8.
47. Parsaik AK, Singh B, Altayar O, et al. Midodrine for orthostatic hypotension: a systematic review and meta-analysis of clinical trials. J Gen Intern Med 2013;28(11):1496–503.

48. Hurst GC, Somerville KT, Alloway RR, et al. Preliminary experience with midodrine in kidney/pancreas transplant patients with orthostatic hypotension. Clin Transplant 2000;14(1):42–7.
49. Alhamad T, Brennan DC, Brifkani Z, et al. Pretransplant midodrine use: a newly identified risk marker for complications after kidney transplantation. Transplantation 2016;100(5):1086–93.
50. Galazka Z, Grochowiecki T, Jakimowicz T, et al. Is severe atherosclerosis in the aortoiliac region a contraindication for kidney transplantation? Transplant Proc 2011;43(8):2908–10.
51. Coosemans W, Nevelsteen A, Pirenne J, et al. Renal transplantation in patients with a vascular aortoiliac prosthesis. Transplant Proc 1999;31(4):1925–7.
52. Wilson CH, Rix DA, Manas DM. Routine intraoperative ureteric stenting for kidney transplant recipients. Cochrane Database Syst Rev 2013;(6):CD004925.
53. Damiano G, Maione C, Maffongelli A, et al. Renal allograft compartment syndrome: is it possible to prevent? Transplant Proc 2016;48(2):340–3.
54. Rouviere O, Berger P, Béziat C, et al. Acute thrombosis of renal transplant artery: graft salvage by means of intra-arterial fibrinolysis. Transplantation 2002;73(3):403–9.
55. Humar A, Key N, Ramcharan T, et al. Kidney retransplants after initial graft loss to vascular thrombosis. Clin Transplant 2001;15(1):6–10.
56. Beecroft JR, Rajan DK, Clark TW, et al. Transplant renal artery stenosis: outcome after percutaneous intervention. J Vasc Interv Radiol 2004;15(12):1407–13.
57. Haberal M, Aybasti N, Gülay H, et al. Complete renal vein disruption following transplantation. Transpl Int 1988;1(3):178–9.
58. Veroux P, Veroux M, Puliatti C. Complete renal vein disruption during living kidney transplantation: successful repair with spiral vein graft. Surgery 2003;134(3):511–2.
59. Beckingham IJ, Nicholson ML, Bell PR. Analysis of factors associated with complications following renal transplant needle core biopsy. Br J Urol 1994;73(1):13–5.
60. Pappas P, Constantinides C, Leonardou P, et al. Biopsy-related hemorrhage of renal allografts treated by percutaneous superselective segmental renal artery embolization. Transplant Proc 2006;38(5):1375–8.
61. Ram Reddy C, Ram R, Swarnalatha G, et al. "True" mycotic aneurysm of the anastomotic site of the renal allograft artery. Exp Clin Transplant 2012;10(4):398–402.
62. Kotagiri P, Chembolli D, Ryan J, et al. Urinary tract infections in the first year post-kidney transplantation: potential benefits of treating asymptomatic bacteriuria. Transplant Proc 2017;49(9):2070–5.
63. Hamouda M, Sharma A, Halawa A. Urine leak after kidney transplant: a review of the literature. Exp Clin Transplant 2018;16(1):90–5.
64. Sfakianakis GN, Sfakianaki E, Georgiou M, et al. A renal protocol for all ages and all indications: mercapto-acetyl-triglycine (MAG3) with simultaneous injection of furosemide (MAG3-F0): a 17-year experience. Semin Nucl Med 2009;39(3):156–73.
65. Farr A, Györi G, Mühlbacher F, et al. Gender has no influence on VUR rates after renal transplantation. Transpl Int 2014;27(11):1152–8.
66. Lubetzky M, Ajaimy M, Kamal L, et al. Kidney transplant complications from undiagnosed benign prostatic hypertrophy. Clin Transplant 2015;29(6):539–42.
67. Linder A, Leach GE, Raz S. Augmentation cystoplasty in the treatment of neurogenic bladder dysfunction. J Urol 1983;129(3):491–3.

68. Kim S, Choi K, Huh K, et al. THE significance of post-transplant microscopic hematuria in renal transplant patient. Transplantation 2004;78(2):249–50.
69. Becker BN, Becker YT, Leverson GE, et al. Reassessing the impact of cytomegalovirus infection in kidney and kidney-pancreas transplantation. Am J Kidney Dis 2002;39(5):1088–95.
70. Green M. Management of Epstein-Barr virus-induced post-transplant lymphoproliferative disease in recipients of solid organ transplantation. Am J Transplant 2001;1(2):103–8.
71. Trappe RU, Choquet S, Dierickx D, et al, German PTLD Study Group and the European PTLD Network. International prognostic index, type of transplant and response to rituximab are key parameters to tailor treatment in adults with CD20-positive B cell PTLD: clues from the PTLD-1 trial. Am J Transplant 2015; 15(4):1091–100.
72. Ramos E, Drachenberg CB, Papadimitriou JC, et al. Clinical course of polyoma virus nephropathy in 67 renal transplant patients. J Am Soc Nephrol 2002; 13(8):2145–51.
73. Hirsch HH, Brennan DC, Drachenberg CB, et al. Polyomavirus-associated nephropathy in renal transplantation: interdisciplinary analyses and recommendations. Transplantation 2005;79(10):1277–86.
74. Nickeleit V, Klimkait T, Binet IF, et al. Testing for polyomavirus type BK DNA in plasma to identify renal-allograft recipients with viral nephropathy. N Engl J Med 2000;342(18):1309–15.
75. Williams JW, Javaid B, Kadambi PV, et al. Leflunomide for polyomavirus type BK nephropathy. N Engl J Med 2005;352(11):1157–8.
76. Arroyo D, Chandran S, Vagefi PA, et al. Adjuvant ciprofloxacin for persistent BK polyomavirus infection in kidney transplant recipients. J Transplant 2014;2014: 107459.

Living Kidney Donation: Strategies to Increase the Donor Pool

Lung-Yi Lee, MD, Thomas A. Pham, MD, Marc L. Melcher, MD*

KEYWORDS

- Living donor kidney transplant • Kidney paired exchange • NKR • Kidney transplant
- ESRD • Living donor • Nondirect donor • Kidney donation

KEY POINTS

- Living kidney donation is an avenue to increase the number of organs available for transplant to combat the ongoing organ shortage.
- Living donor kidney transplants have better patient and graft outcome as well as lower health care costs compared with deceased donor kidney transplants.
- Kidney donation is safe and does not have increased risk of mortality. Living kidney donation, however, has an increased but small risk for development of end-stage renal disease in donors compared with nondonors.
- Kidney paired exchange allows living kidney donation for noncompatible donor/recipient pairs that otherwise would not be possible or require desensitization.
- Nondirected donors and innovations, such as the voucher system, can facilitate donation chains to increase the number of living donor kidney transplants.

INTRODUCTION

End-stage renal disease (ESRD) remains a significant disease burden in the world. In the United States, 703,243 patients were living with renal failure in 2015.[1] Although dialysis can maintain patients for several years, kidney transplantation is the treatment of choice for ESRD. Compared with dialysis patients, kidney transplant recipients have a better quality of life, longer survival, and lower health care costs.[2–4]

According to the Scientific Registry of Transplant Recipients, more than 90,000 adults were awaiting kidney transplant in 2016. Over the past 10 years, this number has overall grown substantially (**Fig. 1**).[5] A shortage of organ availability has limited the treatment of ESRD patients with transplantation. The number of kidney transplants

Disclosure Statement: The authors have nothing to disclose.
Surgery, Abdominal Transplantation, Stanford University, 750 Welch Road, Palo Alto, CA 94304, USA
* Corresponding author. Division of Abdominal Transplant, 750 Welch Road, Suite 200, MC 5785, Palo Alto, CA 94304.
E-mail address: melcherm@stanford.edu

Surg Clin N Am 99 (2019) 37–47
https://doi.org/10.1016/j.suc.2018.09.003
0039-6109/19/© 2018 Elsevier Inc. All rights reserved.

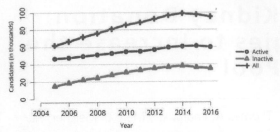

Fig. 1. Number of adults listed for kidney transplant each year. Active patients are those ready for transplant, whereas inactive patients are those awaiting activation. Even though there is a slight decline in the number of listed patients in the past couple of years, there is an overall increase in patients listed for kidney transplant over the past decade. (*From* Hart A, Smith JM, Skeans MA, et al. OPTN/SRTR 2016 annual data report: kidney. Am J Transplant 2018;18(Suppl 1):28; with permission.)

per year remains approximately 20,000. This translates to fewer than 25% of the waitlisted patients actually getting transplanted (**Fig. 2**).[5]

Deceased donor kidney transplant comprises two-thirds of all kidney transplants performed (see **Fig. 2**). There are continued research and modifications to the deceased kidney donor allocation system to maximize the number of organs used for transplant. Despite the increase in deceased donor kidney utilization, the continued organ shortage results in an average wait time of 3.6 years nationally. The actual wait time, however, may range from less than 3 years to greater than 10 years depending on the listing region and patient blood type. Living donation increases organ availability, decreases wait time on the waiting list, and improves graft and patient survival.

Although the total number of kidney transplants has increased, the number of total living donor transplants has remained stagnant over the past decade, leading to a decrease in the proportion of living donor transplant performed (see **Fig. 2**). Donation from a relative remains the most common path of living donation, although unrelated donation has increased over the past decade. Kidney paired donation (KPD), where incompatible donor-recipient pairs enter a registry so they can be paired with other incompatible pairs to make a compatible exchange, has increased approximately 24-fold from 27 transplants in 2005 to 642 in 2016.[5]

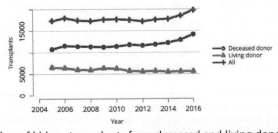

Fig. 2. Total number of kidney transplants from deceased and living donor performed each year, including adult, pediatric, and multiorgan recipients. Although the number of deceased donor kidney transplant has increased, the number of living donor kidney transplant has remained largely the same in recent years. Living donor kidney transplant accounts for approximately one-third the total number of kidney transplants. (*From* Hart A, Smith JM, Skeans MA, et al. OPTN/SRTR 2016 annual data report: kidney. Am J Transplant 2018;18(Suppl 1):51; with permission.)

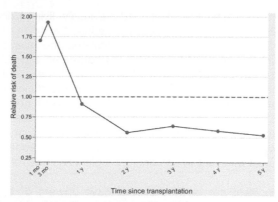

Fig. 3. The relative risk of death compared with remaining on dialysis after kidney transplantation. Although kidney transplant recipients increase a higher risk of death in the immediate postoperative period after transplantation. By 1 year post-transplantation, transplant recipients have better survival than those remaining on dialysis. (*From* Kaballo MA, Canney M, O'Kelly P, et al. A comparative analysis of survival of patients on dialysis and after kidney transplantation. Clin Kidney J 2018;11(3):392; with permission.)

LIVING DONOR KIDNEY TRANSPLANT RECIPIENT OUTCOMES

It has been well established that living donor kidney transplant has superior patient and graft survival compared with deceased donor kidney transplant. In 2016, the graft failure rates for living donor recipients were 1.3% and 34.2% at 6 months and 10 years, respectively. For deceased donor kidney transplant recipients, graft failure rates at 6 months and 10 years were 4.8% and 51.6%, respectively.[5] Patient survival trends are similar. The 5-year patient survival after deceased donor kidney transplant is 86.1% as opposed to 93.1% for living donor kidney recipients.[6] The difference in patient and graft survival between deceased and living donor kidney graft can be explained by donor organ quality, organ preservation time, and recipient health. Living donors are typically in optimal health and free of kidney disease and have minimal risk of developing future kidney disease. Deceased donors, on the other hand, can have multiple medical conditions at the time of donation. Living donor kidney transplant procedures are elective and preplanned, with the donor and recipient operations ideally occurring close together to minimize organ ischemia time. This is as opposed to deceased donor transplants, where cold ischemia time (CIT) is often extended to more than 24 hours, leading to increased risks of delayed graft function (DGF) and primary nonfunction.

Kidney transplantation offers a survival benefit to ESRD patients as opposed to staying on dialysis[2,4] (**Fig. 3**). Living donation, in most cases, enables patients to avoid years of dialysis waiting for deceased donor kidney transplant. In addition, longer time on dialysis correlates with worse outcomes after a kidney transplant. Meier-Kriesche and Kaplan[7] performed a retrospective analysis of data from the United States Renal Data System (USRDS) from 1988 to 1998. This study compared the outcomes of kidney transplants in recipients who had been on dialysis less than 6 months as opposed to those on dialysis over 2 years. Each cohort received a kidney from the same donor. The graft survival was significantly better in those patients who had spent less time on dialysis (78% and 63% vs 58% and 29%; P<.001; 5-year and 10-year survival rates, respectively). Therefore, living donor transplant recipients seem to benefit when they receive a kidney sooner than they would waiting for a deceased donor kidney.

In addition to the medical benefits described previously, living kidney transplantation is more cost effective than deceased donor kidney transplant. Using data provided from USRDS, Smith and colleagues[8] calculated the average payment for deceased donor kidney transplant to be $39,534 compared with $24,652 for living donor kidney transplant. The $10,653 cost difference was largely attributed to the difference in inpatient hospital payment. The average charge during the first 5 post-transplant years was also higher for deceased donor transplant compared with living donor transplant ($280,792.73 vs $223,529.35; $P<.0001$). The cost difference is not surprising given better graft survival and function with living donor transplantation, which lead to less care utilization and less laboratory testing. In addition, minimization or avoidance of dialysis with early living donor transplant has been shown to decrease overall costs.[9]

Living donor transplant has been shown to save upward of 13% at 10 years compared with staying on dialysis.[10] A well-matched living donor transplant provides the least mean cost at $39,939 per quality-adjusted life-year (QALY), as opposed to a deceased donor transplant at $49,017 per QALY and $72,476 for those maintained on hemodialysis. A deceased donor transplant from a marginal deceased donor kidney may have a higher initial expense and a shorter survival but still lowers the costs per QALY ($63,531) than dialysis. ABO-incompatible living donor transplantation, although more expensive at $59,564/QALY, also remains cost effective compared with dialysis.

RISKS OF DONATION

Donor surgeries are under heavy scrutiny. Although donors may receive social satisfaction from the act of donation, they do not derive any medical benefit. The short-term and long-term risks have been extensively studied and found to occur rarely in donors. Looking at the long-term outcome for live kidney donors and their matched cohorts using data from the Organ Procurement and Transplantation Network (OPTN) (n = 80,347), Segev and colleagues[11] found that the postoperative risk of death within the first 90 days was 3.1 per 10,000 donors. In comparison to the matched nondonor cohorts from the third National Health and Nutrition Examination Survey (NHANES III), long-term mortality was similar or lower in the donors compared with the cohorts (0.4% vs 0.9% at 5 years and 1.5% vs 2.9% at 12 years; $P<.001$). The investigators conclude that living kidney donation is safe and does not cause an increased risk of mortality.

A feared long-term complication of kidney donation is the risk of developing kidney failure. Therefore, the same group compared the risk of ESRD in kidney donors with matched control from participants in the NHANES III who were linked to Centers for Medicare & Medicaid Services data to identify those developed ESRD.[12] Of the 96,217 identified live donors, 99 donors developed ESRD in a mean of 8.6 years. This is compared with the 9364 matched healthy nondonors, with 36 nondonors developing ESRD in a mean of 10.7 years. The cumulative incidence of ESRD was estimated to be 30.8 per 10,000 donors 15 years after they donate and 3.9 per 10,000 matched nondonors. The estimated lifetime risk of ESRD for all donors is 90 per 10,000 donors and 14 per 10,000 healthy nondonors. The highest risk was among the black donors and lowest among the white donors. The investigators thus conclude that although there is an increased risk of ESRD in the live donors, the absolute risk remains small. It is vital, however, that transplant physicians clearly convey these risks to potential donors as part of the consent process.

Despite the benefits of living donor kidney transplantation, as many as 30% of patients with willing living donors are incompatible with their prospective donor.

They may be blood-type incompatible or have antibodies against the HLAs of the donor. Therefore, innovative strategies have been devised to address these challenges.

KIDNEY PAIRED DONATION

One strategy for patients incompatible with their potential donor is KPD. In KPD, a pair is matched with other pairs in a database such that a compatible graft is identified for the patient and a recipient is found for the intended donor kidney. In the simplest form of KPD, 2 incompatible donor/patient pairs exchange the grafts resulting in 2 compatible transplants (**Fig. 4**).

More complex matching is feasible with larger databases. Exchanges can be identified among multiple pairs, such that each recipient receives a kidney from another pair. This strategy increases the potential transplants because it allows for more combinations; however, this becomes logistically more challenging as more donors and patients need to go to the operating room at the same time to reduce the chance of a donor backing out.

The development of nonsimultaneous extended altruistic donor (NEAD) chains addressed this logistic challenge and maximizes the impact of altruistic donors.[13] In the past, altruistic donors, now called nondirected donors (NDDs), came forth to donate a kidney to the deceased donor list. NEAD chains, a form of KPD, however, use the NDDs to start chains of transplants that eventually end by giving a kidney to the deceased donor list. Each recipient can receive a kidney before the original donor gives a kidney to another pair. In this scenario, nephrectomies and transplants can be done sequentially rather than simultaneously, because even if a donor backs out, patients will not be in the situation that their donor has given a kidney and the patient has not received a kidney. In addition, the blood-type distribution of NDDs is more similar to the general population than to donors linked to incompatible pairs, for whom it is harder to find matches.[13,14] Based on the OPTN database, 259 anonymous altruistic donors donated a kidney in 2017.

Within the United States, several organizations have developed multicenter registries to accumulate larger cohorts of incompatible pairs enabling more potential matches. These organizations, including the National Kidney Registry (NKR),[15] the Alliance for Paired Donation,[13] and the government-funded United Network for Organ Sharing, actively manage and match incompatible pairs. The NKR is a nonprofit organization that has facilitated more than 2700 kidney transplants since 2008. More than 80 transplant centers across 32 states participate in the NKR. In addition, several single-center KPD programs, such as Methodist Specialty and Transplant Hospital in San Antonio, Texas, and Northwestern Memorial Hospital in Chicago, have also thrived by having focused teams that make matches with more agility than multicenter registries. The San Antonio program has made significant use of immunologically compatible pairs to increase the number of KPD transplants.[16]

The compatible pairs generally have both patients and donors who are easier to match with other donors and patients within KPD registries. Therefore, compatible pairs often can link other incompatible pairs together more easily. Most programs that use compatible pairs in KPD to obtain a better-matched kidney than they would have had had they received the kidney directly from their own donor, thereby compensating the risks and uncertainty pertaining to KPD transplant. These reasons for doing so include a better immunologic match, which results in less risk of rejection and less use of immunosuppression, graft size mismatch, and donor/recipient age mismatch.[17]

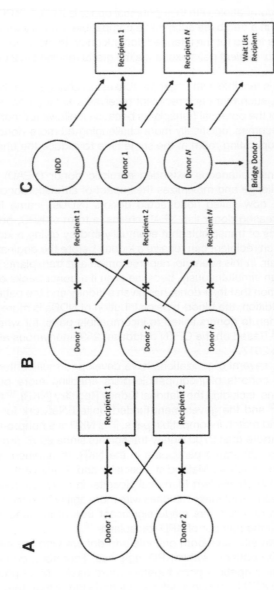

Fig. 4. Possible variations of kidney paired exchange chains. (*A*) Traditional exchange between 2 incompatible donor/recipient pairs. (*B*) Closed chain consists of *N* pairs of incompatible donor/recipient pairs. The last donor would donate to the first recipient to complete the closed loop. (*C*) NDDs can initiate chain donation. NDD can donate to a transplant cluster. The cluster may result in a bridge donor donating to a different cluster resulting in an open donation chain. The cluster may also end with donation to the deceased donor waiting list, resulting in the end of the chain. (*From* Pham TA, Lee JI, Melcher ML. Kidney paired exchange and desensitization: strategies to transplant the difficult to match kidney patients with living donors. Transplant Rev (Orlando) 2017;31(1):30; with permission.)

Challenges of Kidney Paired Donation

Initially, to enable living donor transplantation with donor/recipient pairs at different centers, the donor would have had to travel to the recipient center, or the recipient would have traveled to the donor center. This was financially and logistically difficult, however, for both follow-up and accessing patients' own support networks. Therefore, living donor kidneys are now routinely shipped between centers despite initial fears that this would detrimentally increase CIT. One study analyzed the shipment of living donor kidneys between centers. The mean distance traveled was 792 miles (median 400, range 1–2570 miles) with mean CIT of 7.6 hours (median 7.2 hours, range 2.5–14.5 hours).[18] There was no difference in initial urine output or creatinine decline in association with CIT. Another study compared matched kidney recipients at University of California, Los Angeles, who received living donor kidney either within the same center or from shipped kidneys from outside centers via NKR between 2008 and 2013.[19] Of the 114 transplants studied, the nonshipped group had a mean CIT of 1.0 hours, whereas the shipped group had a mean CIT of 12.1 hours and distance traveled of 1634 miles. There were no statistically significant differences, however, in DGF (0% vs 1.8%; $P = 1.00$), 1-year graft survival (98% vs 98%; $P = 1.00$), or rate of creatinine decline in the initial post-transplant period (-0.30 mg/dL/d vs -0.38 mg/dL/d for first 7 days postoperatively; $P = .11$). These studies have confirmed the feasibility of long-distance matching between centers for live donor kidney transplantation.

The optimal algorithm to match incompatible pairs is one that results in more transplants, better HLA matches, longer graft survival, and decreased travels for involved pairs.[14] One of the most straightforward matching algorithms is the First-Accept Match. Such an algorithm matches a new donor/recipient pair to the first compatible donor/recipient pair that the database can identify. Once this match is identified, the donor/recipient pairs are removed from the database; however, better algorithms may yield better-quality matches for more patients.

An optimized matching algorithm should account for the entire data set and consider the utility and fairness of all the potential matches. This requires computer-based algorithms to evaluate the large numbers of potential solutions. The NKR matching process began by finding lists of the potential of transplant clusters, defined as a group of transplants that can occur temporally close together. A series of clusters form the chains. The chains are started with NDDs. The clusters are linked into chains via bridge donors. These are donors who agreed to donate their kidneys at a later date then the time their recipients receiving a kidney. A chain is considered closed if the last donor donates to the waiting list. An open chain is one that can continue indefinitely. Chains can end if a bridge donor becomes unavailable to donate, at which incidence a renege occurs.

The clusters are prioritized based by various factors, such as cluster length, conservation of group O-donors and availability of group O bridge donors, the difficulty of matching recipients, and quality of the HLA match.[15] For clusters that are equally prioritized, the age compatibility and ease of logistics for transplantations are also taken into account.

Within the NKR, there is a disproportionately large number of group O-recipients and group A-donors and a disproportionately low number of group A-recipient and group O-donors.[20] The outcomes from NKR facilitated transplant, however, have been excellent. In an analysis of the first 100 chain recipients via NKR, 51% were ABO incompatible with their original donor/recipient pair, 47% were crossmatch pair positive, and 2 pairs were compatible but ended up with younger and better match kidney because of participating through the exchange. The mean creatinine at 1 year was 1.3 mg/dL, 1-year graft survival was 98.0%, 47% received shipped graft, and there were no reported DGFs.[15]

Benefits of Nondirected Donors

As discussed previously, NDDs can start a chain of multiple transplants, with the chain ultimately ending in a donation to the deceased donor waiting list. In a retrospective review of the NKD database from 2008 to 2011, 77 chains were identified to be initiated by NDDs, resulting in 373 transplantations in that time period.[21] Of the 77 chains, 4 chains were still ongoing during the study period, 66 chains were completed with a donation to the deceased waiting list, and 7 chains were broken when the bridge donor reneged. The mean chain length was 4.8. Group O NDDs lead to significantly more chain transplants than non-O NDDs. Although there are 40 group O NDDs, of the 373 transplantation that resulted, 133 of the recipients are group O. Thus, despite the chain breaks caused by a small number of donors reneging, NDDs initiated chains still lead to increased numbers of transplantation than direct to the list donation to deceased donor waiting list. Because group O people are universal donors, there are concerns that this would disadvantage group O recipients, because the group O donors might donate to non–group O recipients, limiting the number of donors available for group O recipients. The 40 group O donors, however, led to 112 transplantations of group O recipients within their chain. Blood groups A and B NDDs also led to an additional 21 group O patients being transplants. Furthermore, with these group O recipients removed from the deceased donor waiting list, remaining wait-listed recipients have more access for the available deceased donors. Thus, NDDs benefit group O recipients overall.

Advanced Donation Program/Voucher

Some NDDs may be reluctant to donate because a loved one may eventually need a kidney. Other potential donors may simply want to donate before their paired patient is ready to be transplanted. The Advanced Donation Program (ADP), a modification of KPD and NEAD chains, was developed to address these issues. Veal and colleagues[22] reported 3 cases, where donors were willing to donate before the recipient needs a transplant or even prior to identification of a compatible match for their paired patient. In 1 case, the intended recipient was a 4-year-old child with chronic kidney disease who was not expected to require a kidney transplant for another 10 years to 15 years. The child had a willing donor, his 64-year-old grandfather. Because the grandfather might become too old to donate at the time that the child required a transplant, however, the grandfather donated his kidney in advance to a chain. The NKR committed to prioritizing the transplantation of the grandson should he need a transplant. Essentially, these living donors are NDDs with the provision that their potential recipients will have facilitated transplant in the future. In the 3 cases reported, the advanced donation led to 25 transplants through donor chains. Major benefits of ADP are the flexibility in timing for the potential donors and the reduction of disincentives for individuals interested in becoming NDDs. Once the voucher is redeemed, the intended recipients would receive a chain-ending kidney. For such a system to work, the organization in charge must be appropriately managed with clear documentation and records to enable the voucher to be redeemed and honored appropriately in the future.[23]

Using Deceased Donors to Start Chains

Using deceased donors to initiate kidney transplant chains is another innovation considered in kidney paired exchange to increase the potential number of chains.[24] The idea is similar to using NDDs initiating chains, but instead of NDDs, the initial donation is from a deceased donor to an incompatible recipient. The incompatible donor would then subsequently donate to propagate the paired exchanges as usual.

Using deceased donors to initiate chain transplant could increase the number of transplants by starting more chains, increasing the number of living donor transplants of recipients, who otherwise would have had to compete for deceased donor transplant. Logistical challenges exist, however, to using a deceased donor kidney to initiate such a chain. The fairness of giving a deceased donor transplant to a patient whose family member is giving a living donor kidney away might be questioned. If these recipients are unlikely to be transplanted otherwise, however, they might truly benefit. In addition, some question the fairness of diverting a deceased donor kidney from the deceased donor waiting list to someone with a potential living donor. The utilitarian counterargument is that, when used this way, the deceased donor triggers more transplants and takes more patients off the deceased donor list, benefiting the whole list over time.

Compatible Pair Versus Noncompatible Pair/Desensitization Versus Remaining on Dialysis

For those patients with incompatible living donors, paired exchange is not the only option. Multiple protocols exist to desensitized patients against their potential donors. These generally involve the combined use of plasmapheresis, IVIG, and rituximab to lower HLA antibody titers in the patients such that the crossmatch is negative or the antibody reactivity is below an acceptable threshold to minimize hyperacute rejection.

Despite the difficulty for the highly sensitized patient to receive a transplantation, even one from an incompatible donor after desensitization still provides a survival benefit as opposed to remaining on the waiting list. In a 22-center study in the United States between 1997 and 2011, 1025 kidney recipients who underwent perioperative desensitization therapy with HLA-incompatible live donors were compared with match-controlled wait-listed patients who may or may not have received a deceased donor kidney transplant. The incompatible live donor group had significant survival benefit compared to the control waiting-list-or-transplant group.[25]

Those who undergo compatible live donor kidney transplant, however, still have a better outcome than incompatible live donor kidney transplant. The same study compared 9669 compatible live kidney recipients to recipients who have had evidence of immunologic incompatibility. Those with evidence of immunologic incompatibility had a significantly higher risk of graft loss and mortality at 1 year.[26]

SUMMARY

ESRD remains a significant health care burden. Kidney transplantation is the optimal treatment modality for the patients who are candidates for transplantation. There remains a large discrepancy, however, between organ availability and recipient need. Living donation increases the available organs that improve quality of life, decrease dialysis time, and improve graft and patient survival. Living donation may impart a small increased risk of ESRD development in donors than nondonors; however, the overall absolute risk remains small. KPD and NEAD chains now account for a significant portion of living donor kidney transplantation. KPD innovations, such as using deceased donor kidneys and the ADP, have the potential to lead to more transplants.

REFERENCES

1. National Institute of Diabetes and Digestive and Kidney Diseases. In: United States Renal Data System. 2017 USRDS annual data report: epidemiology of kidney disease in the United States. Bethesada (MD): National Institutes of Health; 2017.

2. Kaballo MA, Canney M, O'Kelly P, et al. A comparative analysis of survival of patients on dialysis and after kidney transplantation. Clin Kidney J 2018;11(3): 389–93.
3. Laupacis A, Keown P, Pus N, et al. A study of the quality of life and cost-utility of renal transplantation. Kidney Int 1996;50(1):235–42.
4. Wolfe RA, Ashby VB, Milford EL, et al. Comparison of mortality in all patients on dialysis, patients on dialysis awaiting transplantation, and recipients of a first cadaveric transplant. N Engl J Med 1999;341(23):1725–30.
5. Hart A, Smith JM, Skeans MA, et al. OPTN/SRTR 2016 annual data report: kidney. Am J Transplant 2018;18(Suppl 1):18–113.
6. Wang JH, Skeans MA, Israni AK. Current status of kidney transplant outcomes: dying to survive. Adv Chronic Kidney Dis 2016;23(5):281–6.
7. Meier-Kriesche HU, Kaplan B. Waiting time on dialysis as the strongest modifiable risk factor for renal transplant outcomes: a paired donor kidney analysis. Transplantation 2002;74(10):1377–81.
8. Smith CR, Woodward RS, Cohen DS, et al. Cadaveric versus living donor kidney transplantation: a Medicare payment analysis. Transplantation 2000;69(2):311–4.
9. Held PJ, McCormick F, Ojo A, et al. A cost-benefit analysis of government compensation of kidney donors. Am J Transplant 2016;16(3):877–85.
10. Axelrod DA, Schnitzler MA, Xiao H, et al. An economic assessment of contemporary kidney transplant practice. Am J Transplant 2018;18(5):1168–76.
11. Segev DL, Muzaale AD, Caffo BS, et al. Perioperative mortality and long-term survival following live kidney donation. JAMA 2010;303(10):959–66.
12. Muzaale AD, Massie AB, Wang MC, et al. Risk of end-stage renal disease following live kidney donation. JAMA 2014;311(6):579–86.
13. Rees MA, Kopke JE, Pelletier RP, et al. A nonsimultaneous, extended, altruistic-donor chain. N Engl J Med 2009;360(11):1096–101.
14. Segev DL, Gentry SE, Warren DS, et al. Kidney paired donation and optimizing the use of live donor organs. JAMA 2005;293(15):1883–90.
15. Melcher ML, Leeser DB, Gritsch HA, et al. Chain transplantation: initial experience of a large multicenter program. Am J Transplant 2012;12(9):2429–36.
16. Bingaman AW, Wright FH Jr, Kapturczak M, et al. Single-center kidney paired donation: the Methodist San Antonio experience. Am J Transplant 2012;12(8): 2125–32.
17. Cuffy MC, Ratner LE, Siegler M, et al. Equipoise: ethical, scientific, and clinical trial design considerations for compatible pair participation in kidney exchange programs. Am J Transplant 2015;15(6):1484–9.
18. Segev DL, Veale JL, Berger JC, et al. Transporting live donor kidneys for kidney paired donation: initial national results. Am J Transplant 2011;11(2):356–60.
19. Treat EG, Miller ET, Kwan L, et al. Outcomes of shipped live donor kidney transplants compared with traditional living donor kidney transplants. Transpl Int 2014; 27(11):1175–82.
20. Pham TA, Lee JI, Melcher ML. Kidney paired exchange and desensitization: strategies to transplant the difficult to match kidney patients with living donors. Transplant Rev (Orlando) 2017;31(1):29–34.
21. Melcher ML, Veale JL, Javaid B, et al. Kidney transplant chains amplify benefit of nondirected donors. JAMA Surg 2013;148(2):165–9.
22. Veale JL, Capron AM, Nassiri N, et al. Vouchers for future kidney transplants to overcome "chronological incompatibility" between living donors and recipients. Transplantation 2017;101(9):2115–9.

23. Krawiec KD, Liu W, Melcher ML. Contract development in a matching market: the case of kidney exchange. Law Contemp Probl 2017;80:11–35.
24. Melcher ML, Roberts JP, Leichtman AB, et al. Utilization of deceased donor kidneys to initiate living donor chains. Am J Transplant 2016;16(5):1367–70.
25. Orandi BJ, Luo X, Massie AB, et al. Survival benefit with kidney transplants from HLA-incompatible live donors. N Engl J Med 2016;374(10):940–50.
26. Orandi BJ, Garonzik-Wang JM, Massie AB, et al. Quantifying the risk of incompatible kidney transplantation: a multicenter study. Am J Transplant 2014;14(7): 1573–80.

Posttransplant Malignancy

Ana P. Rossi, MD, MPH[a],*, Christina L. Klein, MD[b]

KEYWORDS

- Cancer • Malignancy • Transplantation • Solid organ transplant • Cancer screening

KEY POINTS

- Solid organ transplant recipients have an increased risk of malignancy with poorer outcomes compared with the general population.
- Many risk factors are linked to the increased incidence of malignancies after transplantation: type, intensity, and duration of immunosuppression; oncogenic viral infections; and sun exposure.
- Cancer screening is paramount in detecting precancerous lesions and early-stage cancers, increasing the likelihood of a favorable response to treatment.
- In addition to the conventional cancer treatment indicated, reduction of immunosuppression should be considered as part of the therapy.

INTRODUCTION

Solid organ transplant (SOT) recipients are at risk of developing posttransplant malignancy that, along with cardiovascular disease and infection, remains a leading cause of posttransplant morbidity and mortality. Risk factors for posttransplant malignancy include traditional risk factors (eg, tobacco use, sun exposure, history of cancer) and risk factors unique to the transplant population, including immunosuppression, oncogenic viruses, and disease-specific associations. Rarely, posttransplant malignancy is donor derived. Due to transplant-specific associations, malignancies observed in the SOT recipient differ greatly from the general population, and have a more aggressive course. Cancer screening begins in the transplant evaluation phase, and requires continued close attention as part of the posttransplantation follow-up. In addition to the standard treatment indicated by the cancer type and stage, reduction of immunosuppression should always be considered at time of cancer diagnosis with careful assessment of potential risk and benefit. Specific malignancies warrant change in immunosuppressive agents. Early detection and treatment of posttransplant malignancy is associated with improved outcomes.

Disclosure Statement: Dr A.P. Rossi has nothing to disclose. Dr C.L. Klein has a relationship with Veloxis and Alexion Pharmaceuticals.
[a] Maine Medical Center, Maine Transplant Program, 19 West Street, Portland, ME 04102, USA;
[b] Department of Transplantation, Piedmont Transplant Institute, Piedmont Atlanta Hospital MTP Mason Transplant, 1968 Peachtree Road Northwest, Building 77, Atlanta, GA 30309, USA
* Corresponding author.
E-mail address: arossi@mmc.org

EPIDEMIOLOGY

SOT recipients have an increased risk of cancer compared with the general population. Many studies have reported a twofold to fourfold increased risk of malignancy.[1–5] The most extensive cohort study involving 175,732 SOT recipients (58.4% kidney, 21.6% liver, 10% heart, and 4% lung) in the United States showed an incidence of 1375 per 100,000 person-years, representing a standardized incidence ratio (SIR) of 2.1 (95% confidence interval [CI] 2.06–2.14).[3] The risk was increased for a total of 32 malignancies. The cancers with the highest risk relative to the general population included Kaposi sarcoma (KS) (SIR 61.5, 95% CI 51–73.5), lip (SIR 16.8, 95% CI 14–19.9), nonmelanoma skin (SIR 13.9, 95% CI 11.9–16), liver (SIR 11.6, 95% CI 10.8–12.3), vulvar (SIR 7.6, 95% CI 5.8–9.8), non-Hodgkin lymphoma (SIR 7.5, 95% CI 7.2–7.9), and anal (SIR 5.8, 95% CI 4.7–7.2). Interestingly the risk of breast and prostate cancers was lower in the transplant population (SIR 0.85, 96% CI 0.77–0.93; and SIR 0.92, 95% CI 0.87–0.98, respectively), and the risk of cervical cancer was not increased (SIR 1.03, 95% CI 0.75–1.38). These latter findings may reflect required cancer screening before transplantation, early detection and subsequent treatment, and the lack of viral association with breast and prostate cancer. The overall incidence of malignancy within the first 5 years of transplantation exceeds 4%,[1,6] and in one study was 49.3% in those surviving to 25 years after kidney transplantation.[7] Skin cancers are the most frequent malignancy observed in the transplant population, ultimately occurring in 8% of recipients and accounting for more than 40% of posttransplant malignancies.[8,9] Along with cardiovascular disease and infection, cancer-related death remains 1 of the 3 leading causes of death in SOT recipients. In a Canadian study of 11,061 SOT recipients transplanted between 1991 and 2010, 20% of deaths were cancer related and cancer mortality was significantly increased relative to the general population (SIR 2.8, 95% CI 2.61–3.07).[10]

Epidemiologic studies have also found that the pattern of posttransplant malignancies varies according to the organ transplanted. Lung transplant recipients have a twofold increase in non-Hodgkin lymphoma compared with kidney, liver, or heart transplant recipients.[3,5] This may be related to the amount of lymphoid tissue that is transplanted within the lung, as well as the degree of immunosuppression. Additionally, lung cancer was most common in lung transplant recipients (SIR 6.13) but also increased in heart recipients (SIR 2.67) compared with kidney (SIR 1.46) and liver (SIR 1.95) recipients. It has been postulated that this elevated risk could be related to the high incidence of tobacco use contributing to primary pulmonary and cardiac disease.[11,12] Similarly, the incidence of liver and kidney cancers is highest in the liver and kidney transplant recipients, respectively.[3,13]

De novo malignancies in SOT recipients are associated with worse outcomes compared with the general population. Miao and colleagues[14] demonstrated that SOT recipients were likely to present with more advanced colon, breast, and bladder cancer and malignant melanoma compared with the general population. An Australian study of liver and cardiothoracic transplant recipients showed a twofold-increased mortality risk compared with the matched general population (standardized mortality risk 2.83, 95% CI 2.4–3.3).[15] Excess risk was observed regardless of transplanted organ, recipient age, or gender.

PATHOGENESIS

Many risk factors have been linked to the increased incidence of malignancies after SOT: intensity and duration of immunosuppression, oncogenic viral infections, and sun exposure. In rare circumstances, the posttransplant malignancy can be donor derived. Last, for kidney transplant recipients, length of pretransplant dialysis may be a contributing factor.

Immunosuppression

Through the natural process of immunosurveillance, CD4+ and CD8+ T cells protect normal cells from undergoing oncogenic transformation.[16,17] Advances in immunosuppression have significantly prolonged the survival of organ transplants through lower rejection rates. The counter face to this is an increased risk of malignancies through alterations of the immunosurveillance process.

Antibody therapies against T lymphocytes, such as antithymocyte globulin (ATG) and alemtuzumab (anti-CD52), increase the risk of posttransplant malignancies. These agents have been linked to an increased risk of posttransplant lymphoproliferative disorder (PTLD), melanoma, colorectal, and thyroid cancer.[18–20] Increased risk of malignancy is observed in patients treated for rejection within the first year posttransplantation due to the use of depleting agents. The nondepleting agents like basiliximab and daclizumab have not been consistently associated with an increased risk of posttransplant malignances.

Calcineurin inhibitors (CNIs) result in inhibition of interleukin (IL)-2 production, which impedes the activation and proliferation of T cells, the key performers of immunosurveillance. Additionally, CNIs upregulate vascular endothelial growth factor (VEGF) and increase the expression of transforming growth factor $\beta1$ (TGF-β_1). Both VEGF and TGF-β_1 have been demonstrated to play a role in angiogenesis and tumor progression.[17,21–23] The use of CNIs has also been linked to increased production of IL-6.[18,24,25] Increased level of IL-6 can promote B-cell activation, growth, and possible immortalization, facilitating oncogenic viral replication of Epstein-Barr virus (EBV), human herpes virus 8 (HHV-8), and human papilloma virus (HPV).[22,25,26] A dose-dependent effect has been demonstrated for both cyclosporine and tacrolimus.[23,27] Dantal and colleagues[27] studied 231 kidney transplant recipients randomized to receive low-dose cyclosporine (trough blood concentrations 75–125 ng/mL) versus standard dose (trough blood concentrations 150–205 ng/mL). Recipients in the low-dose group had a lower incidence of all cancers (23 vs 37 cancers) but a higher incidence of rejection.

Azathioprine (AZA) is a purine analogue that interferes with DNA replication and inhibits T-cell proliferation. This ability to interrupt DNA synthesis can inhibit the natural DNA repair process that occurs after DNA mutations caused by UV exposure.[28–30] A meta-analysis of the use of AZA after SOT, found a significant increased risk of squamous cell skin carcinoma (SCSC) in relation to AZA exposure versus no exposure to AZA (odds ratio [OR] 1.56, 95% CI 1.11–2.18).[31]

Mycophenolic acid (MPA) and mycophenolate mofetil (MMF) are contemporary antimetabolites that have largely replaced the use of AZA. MPA/MMF block the synthesis of purine through inhibition of the enzyme inosine monophosphate dehydrogenase. A study comparing the effects of AZA and MPA found that recipients treated with AZA were more than twice as likely to develop SCSC (OR 2.67). In contrast, the use of MPA was associated with a lower risk of SCSC (OR 0.45).[29] Other studies have also described a reduced risk of malignancies in those treated with MMF/MPA after transplantation.[32,33] Some tumors have large elevations of the enzyme inosine monophosphate dehydrogenase, suggesting that MMF/MPA may have antiproliferative effects through inhibition of this enzyme.[34] Some speculate that the use of MMF/MPA is associated with fewer episodes of rejection and subsequently reduced need for augmented rescue immunosuppression, thus resulting in reduced malignancy risk through reduced overall immunosuppression.

The mammalian target of rapamycin (mTOR) inhibitors, everolimus and sirolimus, inhibit T-cell activation and replication. The antiproliferative effects of mTOR inhibitors have been described in a few studies. Sirolimus has antiangiogenic activity linked to a reduction in the production of VEGF and reduction in the response of vascular endothelial cells to stimulation by VEGF.[35,36] Alternative mechanisms include reduction of cell proliferation through inhibition of p70 S6K and reduction of tumor cell Jak/STATs activity.[25,35] A meta-analysis of 21 randomized trials of kidney alone or kidney pancreas transplants showed that sirolimus was associated with a 40% reduction in the risk of malignancy (adjusted hazard ratio [HR] 0.6, 95% CI 0.39–0.93) and 56% reduction in the risk of nonmelanoma skin cancer (HR 0.44, 95% CI 0.30–0.63) compared with controls.[37] However, sirolimus was associated with an increased risk of death compared with controls (HR 1.43, 95% CI 1.21–1.71). Increased cardiovascular and infection-related deaths were the drivers of higher mortality in the sirolimus group. Another important factor regarding the use of mTOR inhibitors is the high discontinuation rate due to side effects like mucositis, impaired wound healing, edema, diarrhea, and proteinuria.[22]

Belatacept selectively blocks the costimulation of T cells. Clinical trials showed an increase risk of PTLD with almost 50% showing central nervous system (CNS) involvement in the belatacept arms compared with cyclosporine. This was seen in the EBV seronegative recipients and thus its use is not advised in recipients that are EBV immunoglobulin (Ig)G negative.[38–40]

Viral Infections

Chronic viral infections are well-recognized mediators of specific cancers posttransplantation: HHV-8 and KS; HPV and skin, anogenital, and head and neck cancers; EBV and PTLD, nasopharyngeal cancers; hepatitis B or C and hepatocellular carcinoma; Merkel cell polyomavirus and Merkel cell carcinoma.[41] Oncogenic viruses disrupt cellular mitotic checkpoints causing proliferation and immortalization of infected cells. All malignancies with a significantly increased risk relative to the general population have viral associations highlighting the role of oncogenic viruses in posttransplant cancer.

HHV-8 has been causally related to all forms of Kaposi sarcoma.[42] Nearly all SOT recipients with KS have been found to be seropositive against HHV-8. However, HHV-8 infection alone is not sufficient for the development of KS. The degree of immunosuppression is an important contributing factor as demonstrated by a higher incidence of KS in kidney transplant recipients compared with patients on maintenance dialysis.[43,44] In the immune-competent host, KS is a localized cutaneous disease with low risk for dissemination. However, under states of immunosuppression, KS is more aggressive, frequently multicentric, and commonly involves the viscera.[45] Risk factors include male gender (3:1 male-to-female ratio) and origin from an area with high seroprevalence including those of Mediterranean, Jewish, Arabic, Caribbean, or African descent.

Merkel cell carcinoma is an aggressive neuroendocrine tumor, with high incidence of local recurrence and lymph node metastasis. Merkel cell polyomavirus can be detected in more than 80% of these tumors. As opposed to the immunosuppressed transplant recipient, this tumor is very rare in the immune-competent host.

HPV DNA has been found in 65% to 90% of SCSC posttransplantation.[46] Different strains of HPV have been associated with tumors in transplant recipients, including common benign cutaneous strains (HPV 1 and 2), oncogenic mucosal strains (HPV 16 and 18), and nononcogenic mucosal strains (HPV 6 and 11).[9,46–48] However, the role of HPV in posttransplant malignancy remains to be elucidated, as the virus has also been detected in normal skin of transplant recipients.

Sun Exposure

Ultraviolet radiation and fair skin are known risk factors for the development of squamous cell carcinoma and basal cell carcinoma of the skin, both in the transplant population and the general population.[49,50] In nonwhite transplant recipients, nonmelanoma skin cancers are more commonly located in areas not exposed to the sun and are more likely to be related to HPV infection.[51]

Donor Transmission

Transmission of donor malignancies is a very rare event; however, in the transplant recipient with impaired immunosurveillance, this rare event often results in metastatic disease with high mortality. Donor-transmitted cancers that have been reported in the literature include cancers of the colon, breast, lung, kidney, prostate, liver, melanoma, KS, and glioblastoma multiforme.[45,52–55]

A study of all donor-related malignancies reported to the United Network of Organ Sharing from April 1994 to July 2001 found a total of 21 donor-related malignancies (14 cadaveric, 3 living donors). The cadaveric donor-related tumor rate was 0.04% (14 of 34,993 donors). The overall mortality rate for those developing donor-related malignancies was 38%.[56] Birkeland and Storm,[53] using data from a single kidney transplant center, found a risk of 1.3% (8 in 626) for having a donor with undetected malignancy and a risk of 0.2% (1/626) for transmitting a cancer. A registry study of 22 patients who received cardiothoracic organs from donors with known malignancies found a high rate of transmission and mortality. The transmission rate was 17% for CNS tumors and 56% for non-CNS tumors. Survival for non-CNS tumors was 40% at 2 years, and 50% at 3 years for CNS tumors.[55] Living kidney donors are screened for breast, colon, prostate, and cervical cancer using general population guidelines, and for kidney cancer by predonation imaging. The use of organs from any donor with known malignancy depends both on risk of transmission and the recipients' expected survival without transplantation. Cancers with minimal risk of transmission include in situ and local nonmelanoma skin cancers, in situ cervical cancer, and resected solitary renal cell cancer ≤1.0 cm.[57]

Dialysis

Acquired cystic disease is common in the end-stage renal disease (ESRD) population and is associated with length of time on dialysis. Acquired cysts have the potential to undergo malignant transformation. Renal cell carcinoma (RCC) in native kidneys has an incidence of 1.6% to 4.2%.[58] RCC is most common in kidney transplant recipients (SIR 6.7) compared with other SOT recipients (SIR 1.5–2.9),[3] suggesting that intrinsic renal defects associated with ESRD are at least as important as disruption in the immunosurveillance process.[58]

CANCER SCREENING

Given the higher cancer-related mortality after transplantation and overall worse outcomes, cancer screening is paramount in detecting precancerous lesions and early-stage cancers, increasing the likelihood of a favorable response to treatment. Cancer screening begins in the pretransplant phase (**Table 1**) and remains an important component of posttransplant care (**Table 2**).

Table 1
Recommendations for cancer-free time interval before transplantation

Malignancy	Stage	Pretransplant Cancer-Free Time Interval
Breast		Minimum of 2 y
Bladder	In situ or noninvasive, s/p adequate treatment	None
	Invasive	Minimum of 2 y
Colorectal		Minimum of 2 y
Leukemia		Minimum of 2 y
Lung		Minimum of 2 y
Lymphoma		Minimum of 2 y
Melanoma		
Prostate	Localized, s/p surgical resection	None
	Invasive	Minimum of 2 y
Kidney	Incidental finding, <4 cm	None
	Symptomatic	Minimum of 2 y
	Large or invasive	Minimum of 5 y
Cutaneous squamous cell	Low risk: surgical excision with clear margins	None
	High risk: >2-cm size, >2-mm depth, poor differentiation, recurrence, high-risk location (ear, lip, scalp, temple)	2 y
	High risk as above with perineural invasion	2–3 y
	High risk with local nodal metastatic disease	5 y
Melanoma	In situ: wide local excision	None
	Stage Ia	2 y
	Stage Ib/IIa	2–5 y
	Stage IIb/IIc	5 y
Testicular		Minimum of 2 y
Thyroid		Minimum of 2 y

Data from Refs.[45,66,100]

Pretransplant Screening

Colorectal, breast, and cervical cancer screening for SOT candidates follows general population screening guidelines.[59] Studies suggest that the prevalence of colorectal polyps in kidney transplant candidates is approximately 24% to 33%,[60,61] reinforcing the benefit of pretransplant colorectal screening. The utility of prostate cancer screening in SOT candidates remains controversial, due to the low specificity of the prostate-specific antigen (PSA) as a screening tool, the typically indolent nature of the disease, and the potential morbidity associated with prostate biopsy and prostate cancer treatment. In a study of 3782 renal transplant candidates, PSA screening was not associated with improved patient survival posttransplantation, but was associated with significantly increased time to listing and transplantation for candidates younger than 70 years with a positive screening result.[62] For the prevention of cervical cancer, evidence from the general population shows that the benefits of vaccination against HPV outweigh the harms.[63] Even though vaccination after transplantation may be

Table 2 Posttransplant cancer screening recommendations		
Malignancy	**Methodology**	**Frequency**
Skin	Clinical examination by primary care physician or dermatologist Regular self-examinations	Annual Consider more frequently if high risk
Cervical	Papanicolaou cytology with pelvic examination Cotesting with human papilloma virus for high-risk populations or after the age of 30	Yearly to every 3 y
Breast	Mammography starting at age 40	Every 1–2 y age 40–50 Yearly after the age of 50
Colorectal	Colonoscopy	Starting at age 50, every 10 y
Liver	Serum alpha-fetoprotein and liver ultrasound	Only for recipients with cirrhosis or liver disease and high-risk condition, that is, hepatitis C virus, hepatitis B virus; every 6–12 mo

Data from Refs.[63,101 104]

less effective, it is likely beneficial in this population as well, and should be considered before transplantation if appropriate. Skin cancer screening is recommended, particularly for those candidates with previous history of skin cancer, fair phenotypic features, or suspicious lesions on examination.

Additionally, cancer screening is specific to cause of end-organ failure. Although specific recommendations are not available, screening of kidney transplant candidates for renal cancer is commonly performed per center practice given the more than twofold increase in RCC for individuals with estimated glomerular filtration rate less than 30 mL/min.[64] All liver transplant candidates are screened for hepatocellular carcinoma.

For limited malignancies, such as hepatocellular carcinoma, select lung carcinomas, and unresectable cardiac tumors, transplantation may be a treatment option.[65] In general, a pretransplant cancer diagnosis may necessitate a waiting period before transplantation or render a candidate ineligible for transplantation. Guidelines on recommended waiting times to transplantation are available for kidney transplantation candidates.[66] Waiting time to transplantation may range between no delay to 2 years for cancers with either low rate of recurrence and/or posttransplant mortality (see **Table 1**). This includes treated nonmelanoma skin cancers, and localized renal cell, testicular, noninvasive cervical, thyroid, noninvasive bladder, and early-stage colorectal cancers and lymphomas. Cancers with longer recommended waiting periods to transplantation include breast cancer, malignant melanoma, colorectal cancer, and squamous cell cancer with nodal involvement (2–5 years). Patients with distant metastatic disease are not eligible for transplantation. Limited data and recommendations for nonrenal transplantation candidates (heart, lung, liver) exist; these candidates are unlikely to survive the waiting periods recommended for the kidney candidate. The impact of immunosuppression on risk of recurrence must be considered against the risk of end-stage organ failure without transplantation.

Posttransplant Monitoring

The evidence to guide posttransplant cancer screening is limited, and therefore most recommendations are derived from guidelines available on the general population (see **Table 2**).

Cervical cancer screening has not been studied sufficiently in the transplant population. Recommendations are being extrapolated from the HIV populations and those immunosuppressed for the treatment of lupus.[67] Initiation of cervical cancer screening with cytology alone should begin within 1 year of onset of sexual activity but no later than 21 years of age. Cervical cancer screening should continue throughout a woman's lifetime. Before the age of 30, if the initial cytology screening is normal, testing should be repeated yearly. If 3 consecutive cytology screenings are normal, follow-up cervical cytology should be every 3 years and cotesting with HPV is not recommended in this setting. After the age of 30 frequency of testing remains the same, but cotesting for HPV may be added. Positive results should be treated as in the general population.

For skin cancer prevention, yearly full-body skin examinations are recommended. More frequent examinations may be indicated in patients with a history of actinic keratosis or skin cancer. Due to the high incidence of nonmelanoma skin cancer after SOT, all recipients should be counseled on preventive measures, including reduction of sun exposure with regular use of sunblock and protective clothing.

Kidney transplant recipients are at increased risk of suffering RCC in native kidneys. Microscopic hematuria and urine cytology may not be reliable markers for nonfunctioning native kidneys. Surveillance imaging, either ultrasonography or computed tomography (CT) scanning has been suggested, with a frequency from yearly to every 3 years.[68] A study of 561 kidney transplant recipients found an overall prevalence of RCC of 4.8% but as high as 19% among those with a diagnosis of acquired cystic kidney disease (ACKD). ACKD is a consequence of prolonged advanced CKD/ESRD and affects both kidneys, which tend to be small as a consequence of renal atrophy. Four or more cysts should be present for the diagnosis. Given the additional risk of RCC, the authors recommend more frequent screening for the population with ACKD: (1) Bosniak category I or II: ultrasound twice a year and CT scan if there is evidence of progression; (2) Bosniak category IIF: ultrasound screening quarterly and yearly CT or MRI, nephrectomy if there is evidence of progression even if not reaching Bosniak category III or IV; (3) Bosniak category III or IV: nephrectomy.[68,69] Of note, the cost-effectiveness of this frequent testing has not been studied yet.

Chronic viral hepatitis B and C, as well as liver cirrhosis, increases the risk of hepatocellular carcinoma. However, for most patients, cancer screening with serum alpha-fetoprotein or liver imaging to detect asymptomatic liver tumors is not cost-effective.[70]

EBV polymerase chain reaction screening for donor-positive recipient-negative mismatched patients should be considered in the prevention of early PTLD.[71] Early detection of EBV viremia followed by treatment with acyclovir and reduction of immunosuppression may reduce the incidence of PTLD.

Pretransplant antibody screening for HHV-8 may be helpful to identify those at risk of posttransplant KS.

MANAGEMENT

Reduction of immunosuppression should be considered at the time of cancer diagnosis. In this setting, the risk of rejection should be balanced against the risk of cancer dissemination and recurrence. The decision to reduce maintenance immunosuppression additionally depends on the planned treatment; for example, maintenance immunosuppression may be temporarily held during chemotherapy and resumed at lower dose posttreatment. Immunosuppression reduction is more complex in recipients of vital organs like heart and lungs compared with kidney transplant recipients who have the alternative of doing dialysis if the graft fails. An automatic switch to an mTOR inhibitor–based regimen is no longer recommended, as these agents have been associated with reduced patient and graft survival as well as reduced tolerability due to side effects.[72] Both experimental data and clinical trials suggest that reduction of CNIs lowers the risk of posttransplant malignancies.[27,73] The decision to use mTOR inhibitors versus lower doses of CNIs should be based on individual cases. Some investigators support their use concomitantly at low doses to minimize their toxicities.[72,74,75]

In the specific case of KS, both reduction of immunosuppression and use of mTOR inhibitors should be strongly considered as the initial step, as KS tends to have a dramatic response to them.[9] KS is highly vascularized and HHV-8 replication depends on the mTOR pathway. The change from a CNI to mTOR inhibitor has been associated with tumor regression.[76–79] A registry study showed that immunosuppression reduction alone caused remission in 60% of cases with mucocutaneous involvement alone and 35% of cases with visceral involvement. As excepted, this was associated with increased rejection rates and graft loss as well as recurrence of KS after immunosuppression was reintroduced.[80]

SPECIAL CONSIDERATIONS
Posttransplantation Lymphoproliferative Disorders

SOT recipients are at significantly increased risk for PTLDs including Hodgkin lymphoma (HL) and non-Hodgkin lymphoma (NHL). After nonmelanoma skin cancer and in situ cervical cancer, which have a more benign course, PTLD is the third most common malignancy affecting SOT recipients with considerable morbidity and mortality.[81] NHL is the major hematologic malignancy in SOT recipients, with risk 5-fold to 15-fold higher than the general population.[82] PTLD incidence varies by organ transplanted (intestinal >> heart, lung > liver, kidney), which may reflect both the amount of lymphoid tissue within the allograft and intensity of immunosuppression required. Donor to recipient EBV seromismatch (D+/R−) and EBV seronegative status are strongly associated with PTLD development, highlighting the role of EBV as an oncogenic virus. Other risk factors include degree of T-cell immunosuppression, time posttransplantation, recipient age, and ethnicity.[1] Early PTLD refers to malignancy occurring within the first 1 to 2 years posttransplantation and is commonly EBV positive, whereas the incidence of late PTLD peaks at 10 years posttransplantation with a higher proportion of EBV-negative cases.[83] SRTR registry data show a 5-year incidence ranging between 0.7% and 9.0% after SOT.[84]

The type, intensity, and duration of immunosuppression have been associated with PTLD. Increased incidence of PTLD was associated with the use and dose of monoclonal antibody OKT3, an earlier induction agent that is no longer used.[19,85] Data on the other depleting induction agents (ATG, alemtuzumab) have shown variable associations with PTLD.[85–87] Despite its anti-EBV proliferation effects in vivo, the de novo use of sirolimus has not been associated with decreased PTLD risk and, in fact, may be associated with higher risk based on registry data.[87] Belatacept, a fusion CTLA4-Ig protein that blocks the costimulation pathway, increases the risk of PTLD, particularly in the CNS, and is contraindicated for use in EBV seronegative kidney recipients. Belatacept has a lower efficacy of preventing graft rejection but was associated with increased risk of PTLD,[88] illustrating that the association between PTLD and immunosuppressive agents reflects both intensity of immunosuppression and specific drug effects.

Posttransplantation lymphoproliferative disorders can be host-derived, commonly a multisystem disease, or donor derived, which is more commonly limited to the allograft tissue.[89] Presenting symptoms are variable, including constitutional symptoms, such as fever, weight loss, fatigue, lymphadenopathy, and symptoms related to dysfunction of affected organs. Laboratory findings may include unexplained anemia, thrombocytopenia, leukopenia, elevated serum lactate dehydrogenase, hypercalcemia, and hyperuricemia. The 2008 World Health Organization (WHO) classification of PTLD is used to stratify NHL and HL after tissue diagnosis.[90] NHL ranges from early, polyclonal lesions presenting clinically as an infectious mononucleosis-type acute illness, to monomorphic, monoclonal disease meeting criteria for NHL in immunocompetent patients. The lymphoid cell proliferation is most commonly B-cell, rarely of T-cell or natural killer–cell origin. Serum and cerebral spinal fluid analysis for EBV viral load, and radiologic features can be used to make a presumptive diagnosis if tissue diagnosis is impossible due to location (eg, CNS lesions). CT and PET can be used to stage and monitor response to treatment.[91]

Screening methods and prophylaxis for PTLD are limited and controversial. Screening for PTLD using EBV viral load in peripheral blood has been used, particularly in higher risk situations (EBV D+/R−), as higher EBV viral loads have been observed in PTLD cases.[92,93] However, several limitations to this screening technique exist, including lack of standardization among EBV assays, significant overlap in viral loads between PTLD and non-PTLD cases leading to low positive and negative predictive values, and lack of utility in EBV-negative PTLD. Some have suggested that the trend in viral loads to be more predictive,[94] advocating reduction of immunosuppression in high-risk patients with increasing viral loads.[95] Chemoprophylaxis for PTLD is also debated, as antiviral agents, such as acyclovir and ganciclovir, do not appear to prevent development of EBV viremia despite in vitro activity against EBV.[96,97]

Treatment options for PTLD depend on WHO classification, B-cell expression of CD20, and location and staging of disease, and include reduction of immunosuppression, anti–B-cell antibodies, chemotherapy, surgery, and radiation. Reduction of immunosuppression is a first-line intervention, particularly for early lesions. Risks of immunosuppression reduction alone, including allograft rejection and failure must be carefully weighed against expected tumor response. More advanced PTLD, including CNS disease, requires chemotherapy. The anti–B-cell antibody rituximab is used in CD20-positive B-cell PTLD. Rituximab is used alone or in combination with the CHOP regimen (cyclophosphamide, hydroxydaunorubicin or doxorubicin, oncovin or vincristine, and prednisone) for more advanced PTLD.[98,99] Results from the multicenter prospective PTLD-1 trial show early rituximab followed by full-dose CHOP chemotherapy in cases with insufficient response to rituximab alone, resulted in 68% complete response, 22% partial response, treatment-related mortality of 11%, and median overall survival of 6.6 years.[98] Given the lack of data supporting antiviral agents for chemoprophylaxis, these are not recommended for treatment, although added as adjunctive therapy by some centers. Survivors achieving PTLD remission may suffer allograft failure with consideration of retransplantation. It is unclear whether retransplantation is safe in a patient with persistently positive EBV viral load.

SUMMARY

SOT recipients have an increased risk of malignancies and increased cancer-related mortality when compared with the general population. Along with traditional risk factors for cancer development, immunosuppression and oncogenic viral infections play an important role in the pathogenesis of posttransplant malignancies. Guidelines exist for cancer screening in kidney transplant recipients; however, guidelines are scarce and variable for other SOT recipients. Immunosuppression manipulation should be considered as part of the initial treatment, while considering the risk of rejection and overall outcomes. Early detection and treatment are associated with improved survival.

REFERENCES

1. Collett D, Mumford L, Banner NR, et al. Comparison of the incidence of malignancy in recipients of different types of organ: a UK Registry audit. Am J Transplant 2010;10(8):1889–96.
2. Villeneuve PJ, Schaubel DE, Fenton SS, et al. Cancer incidence among Canadian kidney transplant recipients. Am J Transplant 2007;7(4):941–8.
3. Engels EA, Pfeiffer RM, Fraumeni JF Jr, et al. Spectrum of cancer risk among US solid organ transplant recipients. JAMA 2011;306(17):1891–901.
4. Kyllonen L, Salmela K, Pukkala E. Cancer incidence in a kidney-transplanted population. Transpl Int 2000;13(Suppl 1):S394–8.
5. Grulich AE, van Leeuwen MT, Falster MO, et al. Incidence of cancers in people with HIV/AIDS compared with immunosuppressed transplant recipients: a meta-analysis. Lancet 2007;370(9581):59–67.
6. Hall EC, Pfeiffer RM, Segev DL, et al. Cumulative incidence of cancer after solid organ transplantation. Cancer 2013;119(12):2300–8.
7. Wimmer CD, Rentsch M, Crispin A, et al. The janus face of immunosuppression—de novo malignancy after renal transplantation: the experience of the Transplantation Center Munich. Kidney Int 2007;71(12):1271–8.
8. Garrett GL, Blanc PD, Boscardin J, et al. Incidence of and risk factors for skin cancer in organ transplant recipients in the United States. JAMA Dermatol 2017;153(3):296–303.
9. Euvrard S, Kanitakis J, Claudy A. Skin cancers after organ transplantation. N Engl J Med 2003;348(17):1681–91.
10. Acuna SA, Fernandes KA, Daly C, et al. Cancer mortality among recipients of solid-organ transplantation in Ontario, Canada. JAMA Oncol 2016;2(4):463–9.
11. Anyanwu AC, Townsend ER, Banner NR, et al. Primary lung carcinoma after heart or lung transplantation: management and outcome. J Thorac Cardiovasc Surg 2002;124(6):1190–7.
12. Goldstein DJ, Austin JH, Zuech N, et al. Carcinoma of the lung after heart transplantation. Transplantation 1996;62(6):772–5.
13. Doycheva I, Amer S, Watt KD. De novo malignancies after transplantation: risk and surveillance strategies. Med Clin North Am 2016;100(3):551–67.
14. Miao Y, Everly JJ, Gross TG, et al. De novo cancers arising in organ transplant recipients are associated with adverse outcomes compared with the general population. Transplantation 2009;87(9):1347–59.
15. Na R, Grulich AE, Meagher NS, et al. De novo cancer-related death in Australian liver and cardiothoracic transplant recipients. Am J Transplant 2013;13(5):1296–304.
16. Dunn GP, Old LJ, Schreiber RD. The immunobiology of cancer immunosurveillance and immunoediting. Immunity 2004;21(2):137–48.
17. Billups K, Neal J, Salyer J. Immunosuppressant-driven de novo malignant neoplasms after solid-organ transplant. Prog Transplant 2015;25(2):182–8.

18. Caillard S, Dharnidharka V, Agodoa L, et al. Posttransplant lymphoproliferative disorders after renal transplantation in the United States in era of modern immunosuppression. Transplantation 2005;80(9):1233–43.

19. Hall EC, Engels EA, Pfeiffer RM, et al. Association of antibody induction immunosuppression with cancer after kidney transplantation. Transplantation 2015; 99(5):1051–7.

20. Malvezzi P, Jouve T, Rostaing L. Induction by anti-thymocyte globulins in kidney transplantation: a review of the literature and current usage. J Nephropathol 2015;4(4):110–5.

21. Engels EA, Jennings L, Kemp TJ, et al. Circulating TGF-beta1 and VEGF and risk of cancer among liver transplant recipients. Cancer Med 2015;4(8):1252–7.

22. Krisl JC, Doan VP. Chemotherapy and transplantation: the role of immunosuppression in malignancy and a review of antineoplastic agents in solid organ transplant recipients. Am J Transplant 2017;17(8):1974–91.

23. Maluccio M, Sharma V, Lagman M, et al. Tacrolimus enhances transforming growth factor-beta1 expression and promotes tumor progression. Transplantation 2003;76(3):597–602.

24. Cherikh WS, Kauffman HM, McBride MA, et al. Association of the type of induction immunosuppression with posttransplant lymphoproliferative disorder, graft survival, and patient survival after primary kidney transplantation. Transplantation 2003;76(9):1289–93.

25. Guba M, Graeb C, Jauch KW, et al. Pro- and anti-cancer effects of immunosuppressive agents used in organ transplantation. Transplantation 2004;77(12): 1777–82.

26. Campistol JM, Cuervas-Mons V, Manito N, et al. New concepts and best practices for management of pre- and post-transplantation cancer. Transplant Rev (Orlando) 2012;26(4):261–79.

27. Dantal J, Hourmant M, Cantarovich D, et al. Effect of long-term immunosuppression in kidney-graft recipients on cancer incidence: randomised comparison of two cyclosporin regimens. Lancet 1998;351(9103):623–8.

28. Harwood CA, Attard NR, O'Donovan P, et al. PTCH mutations in basal cell carcinomas from azathioprine-treated organ transplant recipients. Br J Cancer 2008;99(8):1276–84.

29. Coghill AE, Johnson LG, Berg D, et al. Immunosuppressive medications and squamous cell skin carcinoma: nested case-control study within the skin cancer after organ transplant (SCOT) cohort. Am J Transplant 2016;16(2):565–73.

30. Perrett CM, Walker SL, O'Donovan P, et al. Azathioprine treatment photosensitizes human skin to ultraviolet A radiation. Br J Dermatol 2008;159(1):198–204.

31. Jiyad Z, Olsen CM, Burke MT, et al. Azathioprine and risk of skin cancer in organ transplant recipients: systematic review and meta-analysis. Am J Transplant 2016;16(12):3490–503.

32. O'Neill JO, Edwards LB, Taylor DO. Mycophenolate mofetil and risk of developing malignancy after orthotopic heart transplantation: analysis of the transplant registry of the International Society for Heart and Lung Transplantation. J Heart Lung Transplant 2006;25(10):1186–91.

33. Robson R, Cecka JM, Opelz G, et al. Prospective registry-based observational cohort study of the long-term risk of malignancies in renal transplant patients treated with mycophenolate mofetil. Am J Transplant 2005;5(12):2954–60.

34. Buell JF, Gross TG, Woodle ES. Malignancy after transplantation. Transplantation 2005;80(2 Suppl):S254–64.

35. Guba M, von Breitenbuch P, Steinbauer M, et al. Rapamycin inhibits primary and metastatic tumor growth by antiangiogenesis: involvement of vascular endothelial growth factor. Nat Med 2002;8(2):128–35.

36. Luan FL, Ding R, Sharma VK, et al. Rapamycin is an effective inhibitor of human renal cancer metastasis. Kidney Int 2003;63(3):917–26.

37. Knoll GA, Kokolo MB, Mallick R, et al. Effect of sirolimus on malignancy and survival after kidney transplantation: systematic review and meta-analysis of individual patient data. BMJ 2014;349:g6679.

38. Vincenti F, Larsen CP, Alberu J, et al. Three-year outcomes from BENEFIT, a randomized, active-controlled, parallel-group study in adult kidney transplant recipients. Am J Transplant 2012;12(1):210–7.

39. Vincenti F, Larsen C, Durrbach A, et al. Costimulation blockade with belatacept in renal transplantation. N Engl J Med 2005;353(8):770–81.

40. Martin ST, Powell JT, Patel M, et al. Risk of posttransplant lymphoproliferative disorder associated with use of belatacept. Am J Health Syst Pharm 2013; 70(22):1977–83.

41. Vajdic CM, van Leeuwen MT. Cancer incidence and risk factors after solid organ transplantation. Int J Cancer 2009;125(8):1747–54.

42. Munoz P, Alvarez P, de Ory F, et al. Incidence and clinical characteristics of Kaposi sarcoma after solid organ transplantation in Spain: importance of seroconversion against HHV-8. Medicine 2002;81(4):293–304.

43. Brunner FP, Landais P, Selwood NH. Malignancies after renal transplantation: the EDTA-ERA registry experience. European Dialysis and Transplantation Association-European Renal Association. Nephrol Dial Transplant 1995; 10(Suppl 1):74–80.

44. Montagnino G, Lorca E, Tarantino A, et al. Cancer incidence in 854 kidney transplant recipients from a single institution: comparison with normal population and with patients under dialytic treatment. Clin Transplant 1996;10(5):461–9.

45. Chapman JR, Webster AC, Wong G. Cancer in the transplant recipient. Cold Spring Harb Perspect Med 2013;3(7).

46. Harwood CA, Surentheran T, McGregor JM, et al. Human papillomavirus infection and non-melanoma skin cancer in immunosuppressed and immunocompetent individuals. J Med Virol 2000;61(3):289–97.

47. Euvrard S, Chardonnet Y, Pouteil-Noble C, et al. Association of skin malignancies with various and multiple carcinogenic and noncarcinogenic human papillomaviruses in renal transplant recipients. Cancer 1993;72(7):2198–206.

48. de Jong-Tieben LM, Berkhout RJ, ter Schegget J, et al. The prevalence of human papillomavirus DNA in benign keratotic skin lesions of renal transplant recipients with and without a history of skin cancer is equally high: a clinical study to assess risk factors for keratotic skin lesions and skin cancer. Transplantation 2000;69(1):44–9.

49. Caforio AL, Fortina AB, Piaserico S, et al. Skin cancer in heart transplant recipients: risk factor analysis and relevance of immunosuppressive therapy. Circulation 2000;102(19 Suppl 3):III222–7.

50. Ramsay HM, Fryer AA, Hawley CM, et al. Factors associated with nonmelanoma skin cancer following renal transplantation in Queensland, Australia. J Am Acad Dermatol 2003;49(3):397–406.

51. Pritchett EN, Doyle A, Shaver CM, et al. Nonmelanoma skin cancer in nonwhite organ transplant recipients. JAMA Dermatol 2016;152(12):1348–53.

52. Kauffman HM, McBride MA, Cherikh WS, et al. Transplant tumor registry: donors with central nervous system tumors1. Transplantation 2002;73(4):579–82.

53. Birkeland SA, Storm HH. Risk for tumor and other disease transmission by transplantation: a population-based study of unrecognized malignancies and other diseases in organ donors. Transplantation 2002;74(10):1409–13.

54. Penn I. Malignant melanoma in organ allograft recipients. Transplantation 1996; 61(2):274–8.

55. Buell JF, Trofe J, Hanaway MJ, et al. Transmission of donor cancer into cardiothoracic transplant recipients. Surgery 2001;130(4):660–6 [discussion: 666–8].

56. Myron Kauffman H, McBride MA, Cherikh WS, et al. Transplant tumor registry: donor related malignancies. Transplantation 2002;74(3):358–62.

57. Nalesnik MA, Woodle ES, Dimaio JM, et al. Donor-transmitted malignancies in organ transplantation: assessment of clinical risk. Am J Transplant 2011;11(6): 1140–7.

58. Muruve NA, Shoskes DA. Genitourinary malignancies in solid organ transplant recipients. Transplantation 2005;80(6):709–16.

59. Knoll G, Cockfield S, Blydt-Hansen T, et al. Canadian Society of Transplantation: consensus guidelines on eligibility for kidney transplantation. CMAJ 2005; 173(10):S1–25.

60. AlAmeel T, Bseiso B, AlBugami MM, et al. Yield of screening colonoscopy in renal transplant candidates. Can J Gastroenterol Hepatol 2015;29(8):423–6.

61. Therrien A, Giard JM, Hebert MJ, et al. Importance of pre-transplant colonoscopy in renal transplant recipients. J Clin Med Res 2014;6(6):414–21.

62. Vitiello GA, Sayed BA, Wardenburg M, et al. Utility of prostate cancer screening in kidney transplant candidates. J Am Soc Nephrol 2016;27(7):2157–63.

63. Kidney Disease: Improving Global Outcomes (KDIGO) Transplant Work Group. KDIGO clinical practice guideline for the care of kidney transplant recipients. Am J Transplant 2009;9(Suppl 3):S1–155.

64. Lowrance WT, Ordonez J, Udaltsova N, et al. CKD and the risk of incident cancer. J Am Soc Nephrol 2014;25(10):2327–34.

65. Vegso G, Gorog D, Fehervari I, et al. Role of organ transplantation in the treatment of malignancies: hepatocellular carcinoma as the most common tumour treated with transplantation. Pathol Oncol Res 2012;18(1):1–10.

66. Kasiske BL, Cangro CB, Hariharan S, et al. The evaluation of renal transplantation candidates: clinical practice guidelines. Am J Transplant 2001;1(Suppl 2): 3–95.

67. Committee on Practice Bulletins—Gynecology. Practice Bulletin No. 168: cervical cancer screening and prevention. Obstet Gynecol 2016;128(4):e111–30.

68. Doublet JD, Peraldi MN, Gattegno B, et al. Renal cell carcinoma of native kidneys: prospective study of 129 renal transplant patients. J Urol 1997;158(1): 42–4.

69. Scandling JD. Acquired cystic kidney disease and renal cell cancer after transplantation: time to rethink screening? Clin J Am Soc Nephrol 2007;2(4):621–2.

70. Sarasin FP, Giostra E, Hadengue A. Cost-effectiveness of screening for detection of small hepatocellular carcinoma in western patients with Child-Pugh class A cirrhosis. Am J Med 1996;101(4):422–34.

71. Martin SI, Dodson B, Wheeler C, et al. Monitoring infection with Epstein-Barr virus among seromismatch adult renal transplant recipients. Am J Transplant 2011;11(5):1058–63.

72. Dantal J, Campone M. Daunting but worthy goal: reducing the de novo cancer incidence after transplantation. Transplantation 2016;100(12):2569–83.

73. Vivarelli M, Cucchetti A, Piscaglia F, et al. Analysis of risk factors for tumor recurrence after liver transplantation for hepatocellular carcinoma: key role of immunosuppression. Liver Transpl 2005;11(5):497–503.
74. Kauffman HM, Cherikh WS, Cheng Y, et al. Maintenance immunosuppression with target-of-rapamycin inhibitors is associated with a reduced incidence of de novo malignancies. Transplantation 2005;80(7):883–9.
75. Wulff BC, Kusewitt DF, VanBuskirk AM, et al. Sirolimus reduces the incidence and progression of UVB-induced skin cancer in SKH mice even with co-administration of cyclosporine A. J Invest Dermatol 2008;128(10):2467–73.
76. Lebbe C, Legendre C, Frances C. Kaposi sarcoma in transplantation. Transplant Rev (Orlando) 2008;22(4):252–61.
77. Stallone G, Schena A, Infante B, et al. Sirolimus for Kaposi's sarcoma in renal-transplant recipients. N Engl J Med 2005;352(13):1317–23.
78. Campistol JM, Gutierrez-Dalmau A, Torregrosa JV. Conversion to sirolimus: a successful treatment for posttransplantation Kaposi's sarcoma. Transplantation 2004;77(5):760–2.
79. Lebbe C, Euvrard S, Barrou B, et al. Sirolimus conversion for patients with post-transplant Kaposi's sarcoma. Am J Transplant 2006;6(9):2164–8.
80. Penn I. Sarcomas in organ allograft recipients. Transplantation 1995;60(12):1485–91.
81. Penn I. Cancers complicating organ transplantation. N Engl J Med 1990;323(25):1767–9.
82. Dharnidharka VR, Webster AC, Martinez OM, et al. Post-transplant lymphoproliferative disorders. Nat Rev Dis Primers 2016;2:15088.
83. Schober T, Framke T, Kreipe H, et al. Characteristics of early and late PTLD development in pediatric solid organ transplant recipients. Transplantation 2013;95(1):240–6.
84. Kotton CN, Huprikar S, Kumar D. Transplant infectious diseases: a review of the scientific registry of transplant recipients published data. Am J Transplant 2017;17(6):1439–46.
85. Opelz G, Dohler B. Lymphomas after solid organ transplantation: a collaborative transplant study report. Am J Transplant 2004;4(2):222–30.
86. Dharnidharka VR, Stevens G. Risk for post-transplant lymphoproliferative disorder after polyclonal antibody induction in kidney transplantation. Pediatr Transplant 2005;9(5):622–6.
87. Kirk AD, Cherikh WS, Ring M, et al. Dissociation of depletional induction and posttransplant lymphoproliferative disease in kidney recipients treated with alemtuzumab. Am J Transplant 2007;7(11):2619–25.
88. Vincenti F, Charpentier B, Vanrenterghem Y, et al. A phase III study of belatacept-based immunosuppression regimens versus cyclosporine in renal transplant recipients (BENEFIT study). Am J Transplant 2010;10(3):535–46.
89. Petit B, Le Meur Y, Jaccard A, et al. Influence of host-recipient origin on clinical aspects of posttransplantation lymphoproliferative disorders in kidney transplantation. Transplantation 2002;73(2):265–71.
90. Swerdlow SH, Campo E, Pileri SA, et al. The 2016 revision of the World Health Organization classification of lymphoid neoplasms. Blood 2016;127(20):2375–90.
91. Panagiotidis E, Quigley AM, Pencharz D, et al. (18)F-fluorodeoxyglucose positron emission tomography/computed tomography in diagnosis of post-transplant lymphoproliferative disorder. Leuk Lymphoma 2014;55(3):515–9.

92. Wagner HJ, Wessel M, Jabs W, et al. Patients at risk for development of post-transplant lymphoproliferative disorder: plasma versus peripheral blood mononuclear cells as material for quantification of Epstein-Barr viral load by using real-time quantitative polymerase chain reaction. Transplantation 2001;72(6):1012–9.

93. Tsai DE, Douglas L, Andreadis C, et al. EBV PCR in the diagnosis and monitoring of posttransplant lymphoproliferative disorder: results of a two-arm prospective trial. Am J Transplant 2008;8(5):1016–24.

94. Stevens SJ, Verschuuren EA, Pronk I, et al. Frequent monitoring of Epstein-Barr virus DNA load in unfractionated whole blood is essential for early detection of posttransplant lymphoproliferative disease in high-risk patients. Blood 2001;97(5):1165–71.

95. Green M, Michaels MG. Epstein-Barr virus infection and posttransplant lymphoproliferative disorder. Am J Transplant 2013;13(Suppl 3):41–54 [quiz: 54].

96. Green M, Reyes J, Webber S, et al. The role of antiviral and immunoglobulin therapy in the prevention of Epstein-Barr virus infection and post-transplant lymphoproliferative disease following solid organ transplantation. Transpl Infect Dis 2001;3(2):97–103.

97. Ostensen AB, Sanengen T, Holter E, et al. No effect of treatment with intravenous ganciclovir on Epstein-Barr virus viremia demonstrated after pediatric liver transplantation. Pediatr Transplant 2017;21(6):e13010.

98. Trappe R, Oertel S, Leblond V, et al. Sequential treatment with rituximab followed by CHOP chemotherapy in adult B-cell post-transplant lymphoproliferative disorder (PTLD): the prospective international multicentre phase 2 PTLD-1 trial. Lancet Oncol 2012;13(2):196–206.

99. Trappe RU, Dierickx D, Zimmermann H, et al. Response to rituximab induction is a predictive marker in B-cell post-transplant lymphoproliferative disorder and allows successful stratification into rituximab or R-CHOP consolidation in an international, prospective, multicenter phase II trial. J Clin Oncol 2017;35(5):536–43.

100. Zwald F, Leitenberger J, Zeitouni N, et al. Recommendations for solid organ transplantation for transplant candidates with a pretransplant diagnosis of cutaneous squamous cell carcinoma, Merkel cell carcinoma and melanoma: a consensus opinion from the International Transplant Skin Cancer Collaborative (ITSCC). Am J Transplant 2016;16(2):407–13.

101. Acuna SA, Huang JW, Scott AL, et al. Cancer screening recommendations for solid organ transplant recipients: a systematic review of clinical practice guidelines. Am J Transplant 2017;17(1):103–14.

102. EBPG Expert Group on Renal Transplantation. European best practice guidelines for renal transplantation. Section IV: Long-term management of the transplant recipient. Nephrol Dial Transplant 2002;17(Suppl 4):1–67.

103. Kasiske BL, Vazquez MA, Harmon WE, et al. Recommendations for the outpatient surveillance of renal transplant recipients. American Society of Transplantation. J Am Soc Nephrol 2000;11(Suppl 15):S1–86.

104. McGuire BM, Rosenthal P, Brown CC, et al. Long-term management of the liver transplant patient: recommendations for the primary care doctor. Am J Transplant 2009;9(9):1988–2003.

Liver Transplantation

Patient Selection, Perioperative Surgical Issues, and Expected Outcomes

Erin Maynard, MD

KEYWORDS

- Cirrhosis • Selection criteria • Liver transplantation • Hepatic artery thrombosis
- Portal vein thrombosis • Overall survival

KEY POINTS

- Liver transplant patient selection is a complex decision based on medical, surgical, and psychosocial factors.
- Compared with early reports, liver transplantation has improved overall and graft survival but continues to have substantial perioperative morbidity.
- Ongoing efforts should be made to modify perioperative risk factors to improve outcomes and optimize resource use.

INTRODUCTION

Despite advances in the treatment for hepatitis C, the incidence of liver disease has not decreased and, according to the National Institute of Health, 10% of children in the United States have nonalcoholic fatty liver disease.[1] Cirrhosis carries a significant increase in mortality, with the Centers for Disease Control and Prevention citing it as the fourth leading cause of death of Americans between the ages of 45 and 54 and the twelfth leading cause overall.[2] Liver transplantation remains the only treatment option for those with end-organ failure. In addition to increased mortality associated with end-stage liver disease, patients with cirrhosis and patients with chronic viral hepatitis are at a 20-fold increased risk of developing primary liver malignancies. Although there are various treatment options for hepatocellular carcinoma for those patients with advanced liver disease, liver transplantation remains the treatment of choice. As more patients are added to the waitlist without a significant increase in the number of transplants performed per year, primarily secondary to donor availability, the burden on the system continues to increase. Although efforts to expand the donor

Disclosure: The author has nothing to disclose.
Oregon Health and Science University, 3181 Southwest Sam Jackson Park Road, Portland, OR 97239, USA
E-mail address: maynarde@ohsu.edu

Surg Clin N Am 99 (2019) 65–72
https://doi.org/10.1016/j.suc.2018.09.005
0039-6109/19/Published by Elsevier Inc.

pool and use marginal liver allografts are a large focus of improving access to transplant, appropriate selection of transplant recipients to maintain good outcomes and decrease morbidity should be considered as well. This article highlights the mainstays of patient selection, surgical morbidity, and overall outcomes of liver transplantation.

PATIENT SELECTION

Patient selection for liver transplantation is a complex decision involving a multidisciplinary team. Although there is institutional variation based on past experience and risk aversion, several hard stops to transplant tend to be universal (eg, active malignancy outside of the liver and uncontrolled infection). Beyond that, patient selection is a difficult process that often is the cumulative sum of risk that prohibits transplant more than any single contraindication. Broadly, the process of patient selection can be divided into 3 main categories; medical, surgical, and psychosocial.

Medical Evaluation

Pulmonary hypertension
Pulmonary hypertension as defined by a mean pulmonary artery pressure of greater than 25 mm Hg is considered a contraindication to liver transplantation secondary to relative outlet obstruction of the allograft leading to graft dysfunction. Given the relative volume overload of patients with end-stage liver disease, elevated right heart pressures found on transthoracic echocardiographs are not uncommon. Further evaluation with right heart catheterization before listing or placement of pulmonary artery catheter at the time of transplantation should be used to clarify the presence of pulmonary hypertension versus volume overload before proceeding with transplantation.

Coronary artery disease
Patients with advanced liver disease have a high prevalence of cardiovascular risk factors (eg, diabetes, cirrhotic cardiomyopathy), but many of them are asymptomatic secondary to the unique physiology of the cirrhotic patient. Only after liver transplantation, when the systemic vascular resistance returns to normal, can the true extent of cardiomyopathy be realized, leading to heart failure early after transplantation. Cardiovascular disease accounts for 21% of all deaths after liver transplantation and is the third leading cause of mortality.[3] In addition to increased mortality, there is a higher incidence of perioperative morbidity, including studies that have demonstrated longer hospital stays, need for inotropic support after surgery, and high rates of ventricular tachycardia in transplant recipients.[4] Despite this finding, a diagnosis of coronary artery disease alone is not a contraindication for liver transplantation. Various institutional protocols exist for both acceptance of transplant in patients with coronary artery disease, as well as cardiac evaluation in pretransplant patients. The American Association for the Study of Liver Diseases gave a grade I recommendation that cardiac evaluation needs to include an assessment of cardiac risk factors with dobutamine stress echocardiography as an initial screening test with coronary angiography as clinically indicated.[5]

Age
Although the age limit is variable between centers, the upper age limit for receiving a liver transplant is increasing, with an increase rise in the average age of recipients from 48 in 1996 to 56 in 2011.[3] As our population ages and the incidence of nonalcoholic steatohepatitis increases, more patients are presenting for liver transplantation with additional comorbid conditions including diabetes, hyperlipidemia, and hypertension. Although advanced age is not an absolute contraindication, several studies have

demonstrated age as an independent predictor of mortality.[6–8] Given the significant organ shortage, efforts should be made to identify predictors of survival in patients with advanced age to best use a precious resource meanwhile not discriminating against patients who will do well.

Nutrition

Malnutrition is one of the most common complications in patients with end-stage liver disease and is associated with increased complications and mortality.[9] Cirrhosis is a condition commonly associated with a net protein loss. Reasons for this protein loss include poor nutritional intake, early satiety secondary to large-volume ascites, protein wasting secondary to frequent large volume paracentesis, and increased beta-adrenergic activity leading to a hypermetabolic state creating insulin resistance, proteolysis, and amino acid use of gluconeogenesis. This state of severe protein malnutrition has often been a contraindication for other general surgical procedures, but may be unavoidable in patients being evaluated for liver transplantation. Merli and colleagues[10] examined the effects of malnutrition as measured by the subjective global nutritional assessments and anthropometry on recipient outcomes. What they found was that more than one-half of patients were malnourished before undergoing liver transplantation and the presence of malnutrition was the only independent risk factor for the length of stay in the intensive care unit and the total number of days spent in the hospital. Malnutrition also correlated with an increased incidence of bacterial infections. There are a number of nutritional assessment tools to evaluate potential recipients including body mass index, albumin, subjective global assessment, and midarm muscle circumference, to name a few. Which tool best predicts outcomes after transplantation have been studied and met with varying results. It is likely that a combination of modalities best predicts outcomes.[11] A focus on optimizing recipient's nutritional status in close effort with transplant dedicated dieticians should continue.

SURGICAL
Anatomic Considerations

Traditional surgical evaluation of potential liver transplant recipients involves careful review of patient hepatic arterial and portal vein inflow. Increasing use of liver transplantation in the setting of both hepatocellular carcinoma and hilar cholangiocarcinoma results in a need for arterial reconstruction. Although the incidence is low, frequent locoregional therapies involving wire manipulation of the artery can result in arterial dissection.[12] Also, despite there being no evidence of clinical dissection, preoperative transarterial therapies have been shown to correlate with an increased incidence of hepatic artery thrombosis after transplantation.[13] Hepatic artery dissection is not a contraindication to transplantation; however, careful donor selection needs to be considered. Given the increased need for an arterial conduit in this population, older donors at risk for significant peripheral vascular disease in their iliac arteries should be considered with caution. Also, an evaluation of the recipient supraceliac and infrarenal aorta should be evaluated preoperatively to identify an area safe to place a vascular clamp without increasing the risk of other complications.

Portal vein thrombosis is also common in end-stage liver disease secondary to decreased flow secondary to portal hypertension resulting in relative stasis leading thrombus formation. Several alternatives exist to establishing inflow depending on chronicity, extent of clot propagation, and collateral venous anatomy. These alternatives include intraoperative portal vein thrombectomy, left renal vein inflow in the setting of spontaneous splenorenal shunt, and jump graft from the superior mesenteric vein. Recanalization of the portal vein via minimally invasive techniques with a transjugular intrahepatic portosystemic shunt to maintain patency can be considered preoperatively. For those patients with extensive but not total occlusion of the portal vein, anticoagulation should be considered to maintain patency and candidacy for transplant. An analysis of the risk of bleeding and extent of clot and potential propagation should all be considered before the initiation of anticoagulation.[14]

Obesity

The prevalence of obesity has continued to increase in the United States with currently 39.8% of adults classified as obese. This epidemic has led to a rapid increase in the incidence of obesity-related liver disease and referrals for liver transplantation.[15] In fact, the percentage of liver transplant recipients with obesity increased from 21% to 32% in the periods from 1988 to 1996 and from 2001 to 2011. Although the various studies are mixed as obesity relates to outcomes, the general trend is a significant improved survival of obese patients compared with their malnourished counterparts, but with increased associated complications with regard to wound infections, pulmonary complications, and hospital length of stay.[16] These trends are likely secondary to physiologic reserve in the obese patient compared with others. Body mass index alone should not be considered a contraindication to transplantation, but should be used in combination with patient mobility, comorbid conditions, and surgical complexity to determine eligibility. Given the risk of obesity-related liver disease, careful thought should be given to posttransplant weight loss strategies to mitigate the long-term complications of obesity.

Previous Abdominal Surgery

Although previous upper abdominal operations (eg, open cholecystectomy) were previously considered a contraindication, liver transplantation in the setting of previous abdominal operations including Roux-en-Y gastric bypass are becoming more and more common. Surgical evaluation should include a listing of previous abdominal operations and notation of surgical scars and hernias, given that transplantation in the setting of scar tissue and portal hypertension can lead to prolonged hepatic dissection and increased intraoperative blood loss. No longer a contraindication to liver transplantation, previous abdominal operations in the recipient should lead to modification in donor selection (eg, donation after cardiac death donor or marginal donors) so as to mitigate reperfusion injury and allograft dysfunction.

Functional Status

As liver disease progresses, fluid weight gain, muscle loss, repeated hospitalizations owing to infections, bleeding, and encephalopathy all lead to progressive decreased mobility. Impaired pretransplant functional status is associated with an increase 5-year posttransplant mortality.[17] No strict contraindication to transplant exist; however, efforts should focus on maintaining or improving functional status before transplantation to improve outcomes.

PSYCHOSOCIAL
Social Support

Psychosocial factors greatly impact the patient's course throughout the liver transplant process. From chronic illness and repeated hospitalizations, to underlying mental illness that can predispose patients to self-medicate with alcohol or other mind-altering substances leading to cirrhosis as an indication for liver transplant, to coping with perioperative complications, and adherence to a complex medical regimen in the setting of recovering from a large operation the need for social support is critical to long-term success after transplantation. Evaluation and recommendation by a professional transplant social worker or psychologist is equally important as a the medical and surgical decision making in regard to recipient eligibility.

Recidivism

Alcohol-induced liver disease is one of the most common causes of liver disease seen by gastroenterologists and hepatologists. Yet a smaller number with alcohol-induced liver failure proceed to liver transplantation. The reason for this paradoxical finding is complex, but likely secondary concerns for recidivism and misunderstanding of the role of recidivism on long-term survival of posttransplant patients.[18] Although many centers use abstinence from alcohol of at least 6 months duration as a criteria for liver transplantation, the risk of return to alcohol is more complex than just the alcohol-free duration of a potential recipient. Additional evaluation of family history of alcoholism, previous attempts at rehabilitation, insight, untreated mental illness, additional drug dependencies, and coinhabitants' use of alcohol should all be considered. Although the use of liver transplantation in the setting of chronic alcoholic liver failure has been well-accepted, the role of transplantation in the setting of acute alcoholism is more controversial, especially when it comes to public perception. However, studies have suggested that, with use of strict criteria for liver transplant in this setting, acceptable long-term outcomes with a low risk of recidivism can be achieved.[19,20]

PERIOPERATIVE SURGICAL ISSUES
Hepatic Artery Thrombosis

Hepatic artery thrombosis can be classified as early hepatic artery thrombosis, happening less than 21 days after transplantation, or late hepatic artery thrombosis. The overall incidence varies anywhere from 2% to 9%.[21] Living donor and pediatric liver transplant recipients are at increased risk of developing hepatic artery thrombosis than those receiving whole deceased donor liver allografts. The mechanism for thrombosis is multifactorial, but with surgical technique being the leading cause. Other risk factors associated with hepatic artery thrombosis are delay in reperfusion, arterial reconstruction, high portal venous flow, or allograft rejection. Arterial thrombosis can be silent and found on routine/protocol postoperative duplex examination or can clinically present with an increase in serum transaminase levels or a bile leak. Although significant initial allograft dysfunction is usually not present, hepatic artery thrombosis that is left untreated can result in biliary ischemia with diffuse hepatic strictures.[22] For this reason, patients who are diagnosed with early hepatic artery thrombosis within 14 days of liver transplantation are given priority for retransplantation.

Portal Vein Thrombosis

Similar to hepatic artery thrombosis, portal vein thrombosis can be characterized as early or late; however, portal vein thrombosis occurs much less commonly with an incidence of less than 3%.[23] Portal vein thrombus like other venous thromboembolism is associated with Virchow's triad (venous stasis, endothelial injury, and hypercoagulability), with a patient's with previous portal vein thrombus requiring thromboembolectomy at the time of transplantation and an increased risk of developing postoperative portal vein thrombosis. Presentation of portal vein thrombus varies based on the temporal relation to liver transplant with early portal vein thrombosis presenting with massive hepatic necrosis and late presenting with signs of progressive portal hypertension including thrombocytopenia and ascites. The differential diagnosis is broad with early portal vein thrombosis mimicking primary nonfunction and late portal vein thrombosis presenting similar to heart failure or malnutrition. Hepatic duplex or imaging with contrast-enhanced computed tomography can be helpful to make the diagnosis. Treatment of portal vein thrombosis is also variable from retransplantation in the setting of hepatic necrosis to symptom control with diuretics in patients with a more chronic presentation.

Biliary Complications

In contrast with hepatic artery or portal vein thrombosis, biliary complications, the Achilles' heel of liver transplantation, occur much more frequently in liver transplant recipients, with a reported incidence of almost 30%.[22,24–27] Biliary complications include bile leak and isolated or diffuse biliary strictures. Similar to hepatic artery thrombosis, biliary complications including bile leak and biliary stricture are seen more frequently in patients undergoing living donor and pediatric liver transplantation. The mechanism for biliary complications can be technical but also can be related to donor factors including the use of donation after cardiac death liver allografts. The treatment of biliary complications varies from endoscopic or percutaneous stenting of the anastomosis in setting of the leak or isolated stricture, to retransplantation in the setting of diffuse biliary strictures.

RECIPIENT OUTCOMES

With improved anesthetic techniques and advances in immunosuppression, the outcomes of liver transplant have improved substantially from Dr Starzl's initial reports in the 1960s. Compared with the nearly 100% mortality without transplantation, patients who undergo liver transplantation can achieve 1-year survival rates of 90% and 5-year survival rates of 80%.[28] Although recipient age, donation after cardiac death allograft recipients, medical urgency, and presence of hepatocellular carcinoma all increase the risk of mortality, the results with improved anesthetic techniques and advances in immunosuppression the outcomes of liver transplant have improved substantially from Dr Starzl's initial reports in the 1960s. Although advances in immunosuppression with lower overall rates of rejection and graft loss, the side effects still lead to long-term morbidity including infection, increased rates of malignancy compared with the general population, new-onset diabetes in nearly 20% of patients, and a higher incidence of coronary artery disease.

SUMMARY

Liver transplant rates are at an all-time high with nearly 8000 liver transplantations in 2015.[28] Despite the increasing number of liver transplants performed per year, there is a widening gap of supply and demand on limited donor resources. Patient selection is a complex but necessary process to evaluate patients who will benefit from liver transplant while minimizing futile transplants. Efforts should also continue to focus on minimizing perioperative complications resulting in retransplantation and more targeted immunosuppression to minimize side effects and prolong patient survival.

REFERENCES

1. U.S. Department of Health and Human Services. National Institute of Diabetes and Digestive and Kidney Diseases; 2016. Available at: https://www.niddk.nih.gov/health-information/liver-disease/nafld-nash/definition-facts. November. Accessed July 19, 2017.

2. Centers for Disease Control and Prevention. 2016. Available at: https://www.cdc.gov/nchs/fastats/liver-disease.htm. Accessed July 18, 2017.

3. Donovan R, Choi C, Ali A, et al. Perioperative cardiovascular evaluation for orthotopic liver transplantation. Dig Dis Sci 2017;62(1):26–34.

4. Borg MA, van der Wouden EJ, Sluiter WJ, et al. Vascular events after liver transplantation: a long-term follow-up study. Transpl Int 2008;21:74–80.

5. Sethi A, Stravitz RT. Review article: medical management of the liver transplant recipient-a primer for non-transplant doctors. Aliment Pharmacol Ther 2007;25:229–45.

6. Asrani SK, Saracino G, O'Leary JG, et al. Recipient characteristics and morbidity and mortality after liver transplantation. J Hepatol 2018;69(1):43–50.

7. Olivari D, Mainardi V, Rando K, et al. Risk factors of mortality after liver transplantation in Uruguay. Transplant Proc 2018;50(2):499–502.

8. Sharma M, Ahmed A, Wong RJ. Significantly higher mortality following liver transplantation among patients aged 70 years and older. Prog Transplant 2017;27(3):225–31.

9. Maharashi S, Sharma BC, Srivastava S. Malnutrition in cirrhosis increases morbidity and mortality. J Gastroenterol Hepatol 2015;30(10):1507–13.

10. Merli M, Giusto M, Gentili F, et al. Nutritional status: its influence on the outcome of patients undergoing liver transplantation. Liver Int 2010;30(2):208–14.

11. Bakshi N, Singh K. Nutrition assessment and its effect on various clinical variables among patients undergoing liver transplant. Hepatobiliary Surg Nutr 2016;5(4):358–71.

12. Jung E, Shin JH, Kim JH, et al. Arterial dissections during transcatheter arterial chemoembolization for hepatocellular carcinoma: a 19-year clinical experience at a single medical institution. Acta Radiol 2017;58(7):842–9848.

13. Ince V, Ersa V, Darakas S, et al. Does preoperative transarterial chemoembolization for hepatocellular carcinoma increase the incidence of hepatic artery thrombosis after living-donor liver transplant? Exp Clin Transplant 2017;15(Suppl2):21–4.

14. Kwon J, Koh Y, Yu SJ, et al. Low-molecular-weight heparin treatment for portal vein thrombosis in liver cirrhosis: efficacy and the risk of hemorrhagic complications. Thromb Res 2018;163:71–6.

15. Bonner K, Heimbach JK. Obesity management in the liver transplant recipient: the role of bariatric surgery. Curr Opin Organ Transplant 2018;23(2):244–9.

16. Barone M, Viggiani MT, Avolio AW, et al. Obesity as predictor of postoperative outcome sin liver transplant candidates: review of the literature and future perspectives. Dig Liver Dis 2017;49(9):957–66.

17. Malinis MF, Chen S, Allore HG, et al. Outcomes among older adult liver transplantation recipients in the model of end stage liver disease (MELD) era. Ann Transplant 2014;19:478–87.

18. Gong A, Minuk GY. Predictors of alcohol relapse following liver transplantation for alcohol-induced liver failure. Consideration of "A-D" selection criteria. Ann Transplant 2018;23:129–35.

19. Lee BP, Mehta N, Platt L, et al. Outcomes of early liver transplantation for patients with severe alcoholic hepatitis. Gastroenterology 2018;155(2):422–30.e1.

20. Daswani R, Kumar A, Sharma P, et al. Role of liver transplantation in severe alcoholic hepatitis. Clin Mol Hepatol 2018;24(1):43–50.

21. Mourad M, Liossis C, Gunson B, et al. Etiology and management of hepatic artery thrombosis after adult liver transplantation. Liver Transpl 2014;20(6):713–23.

22. Simoes P, Kesar V, Ahmad J. Spectrum of biliary complications following live donor liver transplantation. World J Hepatol 2015;7(14):1856–65.
23. Blasi A, Beltran J, Molina V, et al. Early portal vein thrombosis after liver transplantation: the role of the intraoperative portal flow after graft reperfusion. J Univers Surg 2016;4(1):1–6.
24. Miyagi S, Kawagishi N, Kashiwadate T, et al. Relationship between bile duct reconstruction and complications in living donor liver transplant. Transplant Proc 2016;48(4):1166–9.
25. Shamsaeefar A, Nikeghbalian S, Kazemi K, et al. Thirteen-year evaluation of the management of biliary tract complication after deceased donor liver transplantation. Prog Transplant 2017;27(2):192–5.
26. Kienlein S, Schoening W, Andert A, et al. Biliary complications in liver transplantation: impact of anastomotic technique and ischemic time on short and long term outcome. World J Transplant 2015;5(4):300–9.
27. Kochhar G, Parungao J, Hanouneh I, et al. Biliary complications following liver transplantation. World J Gastroenterol 2013;19(19):2941–6.
28. Kim WR, Lake JR, Smith JM, et al. OPTN/SRTR 2016 annual data report: liver. Am J Transplant 2018;18(Suppl 1):172–253.

Pediatric Abdominal Organ Transplantation

Christine S. Hwang, MD, Malcolm Macconmara, MD, Dev M. Desai, MD, PhD*

KEYWORDS

- Immunosuppression • Kidney transplantation • Liver Transplantation • Pediatric

KEY POINTS

- Pediatric liver and kidney transplantation is the standard of care for children with hepatic and renal failure or diseases in which liver replacement is the only treatment option.
- Children enjoy excellent long-term outcomes, surpassing that of adult transplant recipients.
- Because of the high burden of cumulative immunosuppression exposure, pediatric transplant recipients require a life-long close follow-up.

INTRODUCTION

Pediatric liver and kidney transplantation have become the standard and accepted treatment for children with end-stage renal and liver disease. Since the first successful kidney transplant in 1954 by Dr Joseph Murray and the first liver transplant by Dr Thomas Starzl, the scope of indications for visceral organ transplantation has expanded as well as the range of recipient and donor ages. The first pediatric liver and kidney transplants, simultaneous multivisceral transplants, living-donor and donation-after-cardiac-death organs have evolved rapidly into the standard of care for end-stage renal and liver failures in children and adults.

Challenges unique to pediatric abdominal transplantation include recipient and donor size restrictions on allograft selection, vessel caliber and risk of thrombotic events, and the need for allograft longevity. Medication and clinical care compliance is a well-recognized risk for allograft failure in the adolescent and young adult population and pose unique challenges to pediatric transplant providers.

IMMUNOSUPPRESSION

Although pediatric visceral organ transplantation has had progressive improvement in patient and graft survival over the last 50 years due to advances in surgical and

The authors have nothing to disclose.
Surgery, Solid Organ Transplant Program, Children's Medical Center, University of Texas Southwestern Medical Center, MC B2.02, 1935 Medical District Drive, Dallas, TX 75235, USA
* Corresponding author.
E-mail address: Dev.desai@utsouthwestern.edu

surgical.theclinics.com

posttransplant care, the development of potent and targeted immunosuppressive drugs has been critical in the success of pediatric transplantation. Although the review of specific immunosuppressive agents or protocols is beyond the scope of this article, the advent of drugs such as cyclosporine in 1983 led to an immediate doubling of 1-year graft survival.[1] The development of drug and bioengineered agents targeting diverse pathways involved in cellular and humoral rejection, such as antithymocyte globulin (target—immune cell surface antigens), tacrolimus (target—T-cell cytoplasmic protein), and eculizumab (target—complement cascade), have allowed transplant providers to tailor therapy to specific organs and individual patients.

ORGAN DONATION

Organ donors can include both deceased donors and living donors. Evaluation of a deceased donor is performed by organ procurement organization, whereas evaluation of the living donor is performed by the institution where the donor chooses to be evaluated. The final decision as to accept or reject any donor organ depends on criteria at the accepting institution, and the factors taken into consideration include donor age, size, medical and social history, laboratory data, and serologies.

DECEASED DONORS

Deceased donors for pediatric transplant recipients include both adult and pediatric donors. Transplant candidates when added to the transplant waiting list are registered for both a specified age and weight range for a donor. In general, donors are brain dead donors (DBD or donation after brain death); however, an increasing subset of organs is being recovered from donors following controlled cardiac death or termed "donation after cardiac death" (DCD). The DBD donor is determined to be brain dead by various methods, including apnea testing, assessing for brain stem reflexes, or cerebral perfusion studies. The DCD donor is a donor who has not progressed to brain death. This type of donor is removed from life support and then given time to expire. If the donor expires within a certain amount of time (variable based on the organ and the accepting transplant center), the organs will be procured and transplanted. The use of DCD organs is associated with delayed renal graft function and increased risk of biliary ischemic strictures; thus the use of DCD organs is generally limited to younger donors.

In liver transplantation, in which whole livers or portions of the liver can be used, patients can be listed for a wide weight range of donors. A donor up to 6 times the weight of the pediatric recipient can be considered for transplantation of the left lateral segment from an adult donor into a pediatric recipient. In addition, in pediatric liver transplantation, the use of technical variant liver grafts are frequently used, such as hemiliver grafts (right or left lobe), monosegment grafts (Couinaud segment 2), and nonanatomically reduced grafts, where a portion of the liver is removed (removed portion is not transplantable). If a liver is to be split, the split can occur either in the donor (in situ split) or can occur outside the body (ex vivo split), in which both parts of the liver are transplanted.

Deceased donor kidney grafts generally are from young healthy adult donors to maximize nephron mass and transplant graft longevity. In general, pediatric deceased-donor kidneys from small donors (less than 25 kg) are not transplanted into young pediatric recipients because there is a higher risk of graft thrombotic events.[1]

LIVING DONORS

Living donors are options for both liver and kidney transplantation. For both potential liver and kidney donors, the donors are evaluated by a multidisciplinary team to assess candidacy from the medical, surgical, and psychosocial aspects. Imaging is performed to assess anatomy of the organ and to determine feasibility of living donation. Because living donation is an elective procedure, recipients can be medically optimized before proceeding with transplantation or in urgent cases of transplantation, such as acute liver failure or exhaustion of dialysis access, living donor transplant truly can be life-saving.

KIDNEY TRANSPLANTATION

Kidney transplantation is the gold standard for treatment of end-stage renal disease (ESRD).[2] The first successful adult kidney transplant was performed in 1954 between identical twins in Boston, Massachusetts; this was followed by the first pediatric kidney transplant afterward in the 1950s.[2] Since then, there have been nearly 20,000 pediatric kidney transplants performed in the United States.

INDICATIONS AND EVALUATION

Indications for kidney transplantation in the pediatric population differ from that of the adult population. In children, the most common causes of ESRD and transplantation include structural and cystic diseases and glomerulonephritis.[3] The evaluation process of the pediatric kidney recipient includes medical, surgical, and psychosocial evaluation. Ideally, to be considered a pediatric transplant candidate, the child should weigh at least 10 kg and/or should be 1 year old before proceeding with kidney transplantation although exceptions are made in cases of medical urgency.[4] If the child weighs less than 10 kg, transplant centers will institute measures, such as placing nasogastric or gastrostomy tubes to provide supplemental nutrition in an attempt to improve growth. In addition to patient size, other considerations include the following: if the patient will need native nephrectomy before transplantation, the size of the bladder and options for ureteral reconstruction, and approach to transplantation (intraabdominal vs retroperitoneal). If patients are polyuric, have large amounts of proteinurea, have chronic or recurrent infection of the native kidneys with or without severe vesicoureteral reflux, or if the abdominal cavity size is limited, a native nephrectomy can be considered either at the time of transplant or pretransplant. Pretransplant medical issues that need to be addressed include cardiac evaluation to insure adequate cardiac output to perfuse the new kidney, and risk of recurrence of primary disease in the renal allograft. Patients are evaluated from the psychosocial standpoint to ensure there will be adequate support in the postoperative period to understand and administer medications, follow-up with appointments, and appropriate access to health care.

SURGERY

Approaches to performing a pediatric kidney transplant will vary based on the size of the recipient. The patient will need a central venous catheter (CVC) for central venous pressure monitoring, as well as an arterial line in small pediatric recipients or those with labile blood pressure. The CVC will also allow for administration of induction immunosuppression such as antithymocyte globulin if used. If the child is small, 10 kg to 25 kg, an intraabdominal placement of the renal allograft is the most common approach, although not required. Regardless of the surgical approach, transabdominal or retroperitoneal, the vascular anastomoses of the renal artery and the renal vein will be performed to the infrarenal aorta and vena cava. Heparin is administered systemically as a clamp will be placed on the aorta. Care is taken to ensure the donor renal vein and artery are not too long to minimize any vascular complications. Nonabsorbable monofilament suture are used for the anastomoses. Following reperfusion of the kidney it is examined for uniform perfusion, turgor, and urine production. In small pediatric recipients, it is important to ensure that the central venous pressure is in the 10 to 12 mm Hg range,[5] and the systolic blood pressure is ideally higher than 100 mm Hg to ensure adequate perfusion and arterial flow to a large kidney. In small infants and children, the transplanted kidney will sequester a quarter and up to one-third of the child's circulation blood volume due to the addition of a relatively large vascular bed, thus rapid intravenous fluid administration of colloid or blood maybe required with reperfusion. In addition, vasopressors, such as dopamine, may be used to raise the patient's blood pressure before reperfusion. Following reperfusion, the ureteral anastomosis is performed. In most situations, an extravesicular ureteroneocystostomy can be performed. The bladder is mobilized followed by creation of a submuscular tunnel along the posteriolateral aspect of the bladder, and the ureteral anastomosis is performed with absorbable monofilament suture. An antireflux mechanism is then created by reapproximating the detrusor fibers with absorbable monofilament suture. It is important to ensure that the length of the ureter is not too long to cause any redundancy. A ureteral stent may be placed based on surgeon preference. If the bladder is extremely small, a Leadbetter-Politano (intravesicle) ureteral anastomosis can be performed, where the bladder is opened, a submuscular tunnel is created with the ureter pulled through the tunnel and sutured into place, and the bladder closed.

Some surgeons may decide to use a retroperitoneal approach in the small child when anastomosing the kidney to the aorta and vena cava. If this approach is taken, a right native nephrectomy will generally need to be performed at the time of transplantation to ensure there is adequate room for the allograft in the retroperitoneum.

If the child is larger in size, a retroperitoneal approach can be taken to perform a kidney transplant. Depending on the size of the recipient and the size of the iliac vessels, the anastomosis can be performed to the external iliac artery and vein, as is done in adult recipients, or the common iliac artery and vein, if the caliber of the external iliac artery and vein is not suitable to provide adequate inflow to the allograft. Heparin is not routinely administered when anastomosing to the common iliac or external iliac vessels. The ureteral anastomosis is performed in a similar fashion as it is to the smaller pediatric recipients.

A drain may be left in the retroperitoneum around the ureteral anastomosis if the anastomosis has been technically difficult, if an ureteroureterostomy is performed, or if there is need for anticoagulation perioperatively.

POSTOPERATIVE CARE AND COMPLICATIONS

Postoperative management of the pediatric kidney transplant recipient will vary based on the size of the recipient. In general, effort will be made to extubate the patient postoperatively. From the cardiovascular standpoint, every effort is made to ensure the systolic blood pressure is at least 100, with the use of vasopressors if needed. Central venous pressure goals are 8 to 12 mm Hg. The patient is left nil per os for about 24 hours before a diet is resumed if an intraabdominal approach has been taken for the kidney transplant. If a retroperitoneal approach was used, there is usually no postoperative ileus and a diet can be resumed when the patient is alert and awake after anesthesia. The goal of fluid management, following renal transplantation, is to maintain a slightly hypervolemic state without florid fluid overload as well as avoiding hypovolemia because the transplanted kidney is very sensitive to fluid status and hypotension. Because renal function and urine output can be highly variable in the immediate postoperative state, instead of using a constant intravenous fluid rate, the intravenous fluid rate varies hourly depending on the prior hour's urine output with a 1:1 ratio. Once renal function has stabilized, typically 24 to 36 hours posttransplant, the fluid replacement is changed over to a set rate that approximates the hourly urine output and then weaned as the patient increases fluid intake by mouth. Urine output is closely monitored, and a goal urine output is set postoperatively based on residual native renal function and the patient's size. If the urine output becomes less than the goal, either fluid or diuretics (usually furosemide) can be administered to force diuresis, depending on the fluid status in the recipient. Electrolytes are supplemented as needed.

Postoperative complications can include delayed graft function, primary nonfunction (PNF), recurrence of primary disease, vascular complication, urinary complications, lymphocele, risks associated with immunosuppression, and development of diabetes after transplantation, amongst many others.

Delayed graft function is defined as the need for dialysis within 7 days after transplant. In the pediatric patient population, this rate is relatively low at about 5%.[6] Indications for dialysis can include fluid overload, hyperkalemia, uremia, or acidosis. The decision for dialysis is made as a joint decision between the transplant surgeon and transplant nephrologist.

PNF is a complication where the transplanted kidney does not function at all; the rate for this is less than 5% in the pediatric population.[6] The factors that increase the risk for PNF include cold ischemia time, as well as donor age and renal function. The decision to declare an allograft as a PNF is typically made after 3 months. The patient can be relisted for transplantation at that time with restoration of prior waitlist status.

Vascular complications can include stenosis or thrombosis. Stenosis, depending on the time of diagnosis, can be managed surgically if in the early postoperative period or through endovascular techniques if later. Thrombotic complications usually result in the loss of the allograft, be it renal vein or renal artery thrombosis. The hallmark finding of renal vein thrombosis is urination of forthright blood.

Urinary complications can include leak or stenosis. A leak can be managed surgically or nonoperatively, depending on the size of the leak and the time at which it is diagnosed. Symptoms of urine leak include lower abdominal pain, seepage of urine-like smelling fluid from the incision or increased drainage of clear/yellow fluid from the drain, or a stall in the fall of serum creatinine. The fluid and serum can be sent for testing for creatinine, and if the fluid creatinine is 2-fold or greater than serum creatinine level, this indicates a urine leak, which would most likely be at the ureteral anastomosis. Stenosis usually is diagnosed at a later time, where symptoms can include a slow increase in creatinine and findings of hydronephrosis or hydroureter on ultrasound. Stenosis can be managed either nonoperatively with endourologic approaches or surgically through resection of the stenotic lesion and reanastamosis.

Severe risks associated with immunosuppression can include increased risks of developing cancers, such as skin cancers or lymphomas. However, a recent long-term study of pediatric renal patients indicates that transplant patients are at 6 times higher risk for nonlymphoma and nonskin cancer as well.[7] Transplant recipients may develop diabetes after transplantation secondary to immunosuppressive regimens, which can include steroids and tacrolimus, both of which can cause hyperglycemia.

Other side effects of immunosuppression can include hypertension, tremors, and seizure disorders. Detailed discussion of immunosuppression risks and management is beyond the scope of this article.

LONG-TERM RESULTS AND OUTCOMES

Transplantation of pediatric patients allows for the patients to avoid the stigmata of ESRD, allowing for normalized patient growth, as well as avoidance of cognitive dysfunction, bone disease, anemia, and cardiovascular disease. Transplantation also decreases mortality in this patient population.

The long-term survival of recipients of kidney transplants as a pediatric recipient will depend on the age at which the patient is transplanted. Although young children will do well with their immunosuppressive medications, there is an increased risk of noncompliance and rejection and allograft loss in the adolescent patient population.[8]

For the pediatric patient population, allograft survival at 1 year is 95%, whereas the 5-year survival is more than 80%.[9]

LIVER TRANSPLANTATION

Pediatric liver transplantation was pioneered by Thomas Starzl who performed the first successful transplant in 1967 in a 1-year-old child. The introduction of cyclosporine in 1980 greatly improved transplant success and allowed the discipline to develop from experimental treatment to routine practice for the management of ESLD. Subsequently, liver transplantation has seen improvements in operative techniques, anesthesia, perioperative management, and immunosuppression regimes, leading to expected outcomes in pediatric recipients of more than 90% 1-year and 70% 10-year survival rates.

Indications

The indications for liver transplant are different from the adult population.

Cholestatic Chronic Liver Disease Leading to Hepatic Insufficiency

Biliary atresia is the most common indication for liver transplantation in children, representing approximately 40% of all cases. A Kasai portoenterostomy, commonly performed on children with this congenital disease, will delay the need for early transplantation, allowing for growth and development of the child, thus decreasing the risk of technical complications of transplantation. Regardless of procedural success of a Kasai portoenterostomy, most children will develop progressive fibrosis and cirrhosis over the following 5 to 10 years. Children with failed portoenterostomy procedures who become increasingly jaundiced should be referred for transplant evaluation. Children should be placed on the waitlist for transplant if portal hypertension, synthetic dysfunction, or recurrent cholangitis develop regardless of the presence of jaundice.

Chronic intrahepatic cholestasis syndromes including progressive familial intrahepatic cholestasis and Alagille syndrome are other congenital cholestatic liver diseases that may require liver transplantation.

Acute Liver Failure

One-tenth of transplants in children are performed to treat acute liver failure (ALF). Patients present with the fulminant development of hepatic necrosis, encephalopathy, and coagulopathy, arising within 8 weeks of the onset of liver disease and without evidence of preexisting liver disease (except Wilson disease). ALF, during infancy is often

the result of viral infection or genetic disorder, whereas older children develop fulminant failure as a result of hepatotoxin ingestion or idiosyncratic drug-induced injury.
Hepatotoxicity secondary to acetaminophen ingestion may be treated with N-acetyl
cysteine. Immediate liver transplantation should be considered when patients develop
encephalopathy together with severe coagulopathy and metabolic acidosis. Progression to cardiovascular instability and renal failure and cerebral edema are poor prognostic indicators.

Hepatic Malignancy

The most common malignancy in children treated with liver transplantation is hepato-
blastoma, and liver transplant is the treatment option of choice for unresectable tumors. Metastatic disease is not necessarily a contraindication, although this should
be controlled through neoadjuvant chemotherapy or surgical resection of metastatic
lesions before transplant. Rescue transplantation for previously resected hepatic lesions remains controversial because they are associated with a significantly worse
tumor-free survival. Hepatocellular carcinoma is very rare in children and usually associated with metabolic disease; however, outcomes for liver transplantation for HCC
are excellent in appropriately selected patients. Liver transplantation may be indicated
to treat infants with hemangioendothelioma resistant to medical therapy.

Metabolic Disease

Liver transplantation can be used to correct select inborn errors in metabolism. Urea
cycle defects, tyrosinemia, alpha-1 antitrypsin deficiency, glycogen storage diseases,
and maple syrup urine disease are examples of disorders with an indication for transplant. The liver graft may be used to reverse or control disease in secondary organs
and in monogenic disorders isolated to the liver, cure the genetic disorder. Isolated he-
patocyte transplantation and gene therapy may provide a future alternative for management of these conditions.

Transplantation in Neonates

Liver transplantation during the neonatal period is uncommon; however, acute liver
failure during these first 3 months presents uniquely challenging issues as a result
of size and critical illness of the infant. Indication for transplant is most commonly
due to neonatal hemochromatosis, resulting from gestational alloimmune responses
to the liver, or neonatal giant cell hepatitis. The clinical condition of the infant is
frequently complicated by prematurity, small-for-size, or associated multiorgan failure. Ideally, the treating team will optimize nutrition, cardiac and respiratory function,
and support the infant aggressively to allow for growth and development. Plasmapheresis has been used to delay or even prevent the need for transplantation in neonatal
hemochromatosis. Neonatal recipients generally weigh 3.5 to 4.5 kg and whole grafts
from appropriately sized donors are uncommon. Whole allografts of this size are associated with higher rates of failure and thrombosis. Similarly, larger grafts, cut-downs,
or split-livers grafts all have significant risk for complication or failure. Recipients are at
high risk for bacterial and fungal infection. Long-term outcome is around 30% to 50%.

EVALUATION

The timing and urgency of evaluation will differ depending on the cause of the liver disease. Assessment and trending of hepatic dysfunction and sequelae of cirrhosis
including ascites, coagulopathy, portal hypertension, and encephalopathy as well
as nutritional status and growth are all important in determining the timing of listing

and transplantation. Ideally, the transplant team will attempt to gain as much time as possible for growth and development as this will also enhance overall outcomes. During the evaluation assessment of renal, cardiac and respiratory function is completed with identification of comorbidities or additional sequelae of liver disease. Hepatopulmonary or portopulmonary disease may be a consequence of liver disease and require correction before listing. Renal dysfunction may be caused directly from liver disease (hepatorenal syndrome) or as a result of repetitive acute kidney injury events, and some patients may have irreversible renal damage necessitating dual organ transplant. Nutritional status and growth of the child are progressively impaired by worsening liver disease. Failure to grow despite maximal nutritional support is an indicator of need for transplant. Neurodevelopment is tracked over time and is especially important in specific metabolic syndromes that lead to severe cerebral injury. Psychosocial assessment by a specialized transplant social worker is required to provide understanding of resources and support the patient and family have and to identify anticipated deficiencies at the time of transplant and afterward. This should be addressed before transplantation where possible.

CONTRAINDICATIONS

Severe cardiac or pulmonary dysfunction either secondary to liver disease or as a coexisting condition may prevent transplantation unless corrected. Poor quality of life expected following transplantation especially in conditions also affecting neurologic function may contraindicate transplantation. Systemic infection is a relative contraindication for transplantation, and transplant should be delayed where possible until treated.

WAITLIST AND PEDIATRIC END-STAGE LIVER DISEASE

The decision to transplant is made by a multidisciplinary team of providers including surgeons, hepatologists, anesthesiologists, as well as social worker and dietician.

The pediatric end-stage liver disease (PELD) score is the agreed method for calculating severity of illness and is used for organ allocation in children younger than 12 years. Many children will develop complications from their liver disease not directly accounted for in the PELD calculation and centers frequently petition regional review boards for additional priority. The wait list mortality rates for pediatric liver transplantation are slowly improving but remain high especially in children younger than 2 years:

PELD Score = (0.4336 [age]) − 0.687 loge [albumin g/dL] + 0.480 loge [total bilirubin mg/dL] + 1.857 loge [international normalized ratio (INR)] + 0.667 [growth failure] age <1 year, score = 1; age >1 year, score = 0; growth failure: 2 standard deviations less than the mean for age, score = 1; ≤2 standard deviations less than the mean for age, score = 0.

SURGERY

The donor surgeon ideally should be familiar with the recipient, especially in cases where there is a size discrepancy or other anatomic anomaly. Many children will have an existing portoenterostomy complicating the explant surgery and particularly dissection in the porta. This should be factored into the timing of the donor procedure and aortic cross-clamp to avoid excessively long cold ischemia time. Reconstruction of aortic or portal inflow is more common in young children and additional donor vessels should be carefully procured with this in mind.

A bilateral subcostal incision with a midline extension to the xiphoid is used for the recipient surgery. The portal structures are carefully dissected high in the hilum near the liver to maximize length of the vessels for reconstruction. Frequently, a Roux-en-Y portoenterostomy is already present, and this can be used for biliary reconstruction if sufficient bowel length is preserved. The technique of implantation differs depending on the size of the child.

In the infant and neonate a bicaval technique is almost exclusively used, whereas piggyback may be used in older children. Total caval clamp is well tolerated in pediatric recipients and veno-venous bypass is rarely required to manage hemodynamic issues. Important consideration should be given to the need for growth and expansion of the liver with growth of the child. The bicaval approach is more favorable and reduces the risk of future venous outlet obstruction. Some surgeons advocate the use of absorbable monofilament suture (eg, polydioxanone suture) that can degrade over time and not constrict venous anastomosis growth over time. Portal inflow is often challenging in young children with biliary atresia and dissection to the level of the confluence of superior mesenteric and portal veins or venous conduit from the superior mesenteric vein is often necessary.

Children under 25 kg or those in which a Roux-en-Y is already present undergo biliary reconstruction using a hepaticojejunostomy approach. Primary choledochocholedochostomy may be done in older children.

Occasionally it is necessary to apply a temporary closure device or use mesh when larger grafts relative to the recipient are used. Remodeling of the allograft over the subsequent 2 to 3 weeks will cause it to decrease to size appropriate for the recipient.

The frequency of pediatric deceased donors is significantly less than adult donors, thus the use of whole liver grafts in pediatric recipients is limited. In order to use donor grafts from adult or larger donors in younger children, several surgical techniques have been developed.

Reduced-Size Liver Transplantation

Bismuth first described reduced-sized liver transplantation technique in which the donor liver, based on its segmental anatomy, is reduced in size to better fit the recipient. The vascular and biliary system of the remnant graft must be carefully identified and preserved and this is done during back table preparation by the transplant team.

In-Situ and Ex-Vivo Split

Liver allograft splitting has developed as a method to increase the number of grafts available for small pediatric recipients while also contributing the remaining liver for use in a second patient. Techniques have been perfected to perform this split both in-vivo and ex-vivo. The choice of technique type will depend on the donor environment and donor stability as well. The allograft's vascular and biliary anatomy is carefully defined before any parenchymal transection with the goal to provide both halves with appropriate inflow to allow for safe implantation.

Living-Donor Liver Transplantation

Strong and colleagues reported the first successful left lateral segment living-donor pediatric transplant in 1989. Living-donor grafts represent approximately 10% of pediatric transplants in the United States. It is especially well suited for recipients in the 10 to 25 kg range where the left lateral segment is sufficient; however, surgical techniques are available to use the right or monosegment grafts for larger or smaller recipients, respectively. Implantation requires reconstruction of vascular and biliary flow. In addition, living donor recipients benefit from optimized timing of transplantation.

POSTOPERATIVE CARE AND COMPLICATIONS

Posttransplant care can be divided into 3 phases: (1) pediatric intensive care unit (PICU) care, (2) transplant/surgical care, and (3) long-term outpatient care. Immediately following surgery the patient is cared for in the PICU where they typically are weaned from ventilator and circulatory support over the initial 24 to 48 hours. During this time the liver function is closely monitored by repeat measurements of synthetic function. INR, transaminase levels, lactate all reflect the early allograft function. Bleeding or thrombosis is most common during this period and the recipients are monitored closely. High-dose immunosuppression initiated during surgery is continued. Patients may develop acute kidney injury secondary to reperfusion injury or hemodynamic instability and require dialysis during this period. Once the child no longer requires support they can be transferred to surgical floor care where the goals are transitioned to establishment of maintenance immunosuppression regime, resumption of diet, ambulation and monitoring for infection, rejection, and allograft function. Tacrolimus is given as part of the immunosuppression regime and drug doses titrated to achieve trough levels between 8 and 12. Before discharge, the child's care providers must be appropriately educated in administration of transplant medications and familiarized with common problems that may be encountered at home. Once discharged, the child is reviewed frequently in the transplant clinic to monitor allograft function, immunosuppression medications, and for infectious and other complications.

Primary Nonfunction

PNF is rare and characterized by failure of the allograft after implantation. It complicates 1% to 2% of whole organ transplants and 4% to 10% of split-liver procedures. Immediate retransplantation is required.

Hepatic Artery Thrombosis

The overall risk of hepatic artery thrombosis (HAT) is approximately 8% in children and increased in small recipient age, complex vascular anatomy, portal hyperperfusion, and recipient hypercoagulopathy. HAT is detected using doppler ultrasound and confirmed with contrast imaging or surgical exploration. Early posttransplant HAT may lead to fulminant graft failure or biliary necrosis and ischemic cholangiopathy and should be explored and arterial inflow reestablished if possible. Retransplantation is often necessary. Late HAT (>30 days) is more indolent and may lead to slow progressive bile duct injury.

Portal Vein Thrombosis

Portal vein thrombosis complicates 5% to 10% of transplants and is most commonly associated with hypoplastic portal veins found in biliary atresia. Portal vein thrombectomy and anastomotic revision can be done if occurring early posttransplant or if later venography and percutaneous venoplasty is preferable.

Hepatic Outflow Obstruction

Hepatic outflow obstruction occurs in 2% to 4% of transplants present with inferior vena cava (IVC) compression leading to liver dysfunction, ascites, and lower extremity edema. Hepatic vein and IVC venography with pressure measurements will allow diagnosis and percutaneous venoplasty and stenting are best options for management.

Biliary Complications

Biliary complications affect 15% to 20% pediatric liver transplants and may develop as leaks or stricture. Surgical technique or biliary tree ischemia secondary to hepatic artery thrombosis underly most biliary complications. Endoscopic or transhepatic cannulation of the biliary system will allow visualization of the problem and frequently may be used to treat leaks or strictures. Failure of nonoperative treatment will require surgical intervention with creation or revision of a hepaticojejunostomy.

Rejection

Biopsy-proven rejection is diagnosed in 20% to 50% of children and is often suspected with allograft dysfunction and elevated bilirubin, alkaline phosphatase, and transaminase levels. Histologic findings most commonly indicate T cell–mediated acute cellular rejection; however, antibody-mediated rejection may also occur. Treatment of acute cellular rejection involves cell depletion therapies using steroid or T-cell depleting biologic agents. Antibody-mediated rejection may require plasmapheresis, B-cell depleting agents, and/or intravenous immunoglobulin in addition.

Chronic rejection occurs in less than 10% of children and progresses to graft loss if unresponsive to immunosuppression changes. Retransplantation is often required. Medication noncompliance or poor bioavailability often underlies chronic rejection.

Infection

Depending on the timing after transplant the immunosuppressed recipient is vulnerable to a variety of different bacteria, fungal, or viral infections. The transplant team must balance rejection and infection risk in each individual recipient, and patients needing increased immunosuppression to treat acute rejection episodes are at increased risk for infection. Patients are routinely treated with prophylaxis against cytomegalovirus and fungal risks for 3 to 6 months after transplant.

Renal Dysfunction and Complications of Transplant Medications

The combination of multiple agents has reduced dose requirements for individual immunosuppression agents and hence toxicity. The most common long-term negative effect of calcineurin inhibitors is renal dysfunction and chronic renal disease. Consequently, many transplant programs utilize calcineurin-inhibitor sparing or minimization regimens to reduce the long-term impact on renal function.

Posttransplant Lymphoproliferative Disorders

Primary infection with Epstein–Barr virus is a significant problem and increases the subsequent risk of development of posttransplant lymphoproliferative disorders (PTLD). The risk of PTLD is 4.5% at 5 years after transplant. Initial management of patients with PTLD involves reduction of immunosuppression. Anti-CD20, chemotherapy, and surgical debulking or resection may all be necessary in cases where there is failure to respond.

Retransplantation

Historically, approximately 25% of pediatric recipients will undergo retransplantation and most of these will be required within the first year. The most common reasons for early retransplant are HAT and PNF. Survival after retransplant is significantly lower than initial transplant.

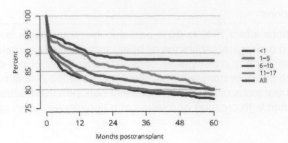

Fig. 1. Graft survival in pediatric recipients. (*Data from* Kim WR, Lake JR, Smith JM, et al. OPTN/SRTR 2016 annual data report: liver. Am J Transplant 2018;18 (S1):172–253.)

LONG-TERM RESULTS AND OUTCOMES

Graft and patient survival after pediatric liver transplantation continues to improve and most recent OPTN data indicate that graft failure occurred in 8.9% at 6 months and in 10.5% at 1 year among deceased donor liver transplants performed in 2015 and in 16.1% at 3 years for transplants performed in 2013. Average 5-year graft survival in pediatric recipients was 80% (**Fig. 1**).[10]

SUMMARY

Pediatric liver and kidney transplantation is the standard of care for children with hepatic and renal failure or diseases in which liver replacement is the only treatment option. Children enjoy excellent long-term outcomes, surpassing that of adult transplant recipients; however, because of high burden of cumulative immunosuppression exposure, pediatric transplant recipients require life-long close follow-up.

REFERENCES

1. Benfield MR, McDonald RA, Bartosh S, et al. Changing trends in pediatric transplantation: 2001 annual report of the North American Pediatric Renal Transplant Cooperative Study. Pediatr Transplant 2003;7(4):321–35.
2. McDonald SP, Craig JC, Australian and New Zealand Paediatric Nephrology Association. Long-term survival of children with end-stage renal disease. N Engl J Med 2004;350(26):2654–62.
3. Verghese PS. Pediatric kidney transplantation: a historical review. Pediatr Res 2017;81:259–64.
4. U.S. renal data system. USRDS 2011 annual data report: atlas of chronic kidney disease and end-stage renal disease in the United States. Bethesda (MD): National Institutes of Health, National Institute of Diabetes and Digestive Kidney Diseases; 2011. Available at: http://www.usrds.org/atlas11.aspx.
5. Winterberg P, Warshaw B. Renal transplantation in children. Kidney transplantation - principles and practice. 7th edition. Oxford: Elsevier; 2013.
6. Salvatierra O Jr, Singh T, Shifrin R, et al. Successful transplantation of adult-sized kidneys into infants requires maintenance of high aortic blood flow. Transplantation 1998;66:819–23.
7. Serrano OK, Bangdiwala AS, Vock DM, et al. Post-transplant malignancy after pediatric kidney transplantation: retrospective analysis of incidence and risk factors in 884 patients recieiving transplants between 1963 and 2015 at the University of Minnesota. J Surg Res 2017;225:181–93.

8. Van Arendonk KJ, Boyarsky BJ, Orandi BJ, et al. National trends over 25 years in pediatric kidney transplant outcomes. Pediatrics 2014;133:594–601.

9. Dobbels F, Ruppar T, De Geest S, et al. Adherence to the immunosuppressive regimen in pediatric kidney transplant recipients: a systematic review. Pediatr Transplant 2010;14:603–13.

10. Kim WR, Lake JR, Smith JM, et al. OPTN/SRTR 2016 annual data report: liver. Am J Transplant 2018;18(S1):172–253.

Pancreas Transplantation
Indications, Techniques, and Outcomes

Mariya L. Samoylova, MD, MAS[a], Deeplaxmi Borle, MD[b],
Kadiyala V. Ravindra, MBBS[c],*

KEYWORDS

- Pancreas transplantation • Islet cell transplantation • Surgical technique
- Vascular reconstruction • Outcomes

KEY POINTS

- Pancreas transplantation treats insulin-dependent diabetes with or without concurrent end-stage renal disease.
- Technique variations of pancreas implantation include portal versus systemic vascular drainage and jejunal versus duodenal versus bladder exocrine drainage.
- Complications are most frequently technical in the first year and become immunologic thereafter.
- Pancreas graft rejection is challenging to diagnose and is treated selectively.
- Islet cell transplantation currently has inferior outcomes to whole-organ pancreas transplant.

OVERVIEW

The first human pancreas transplant was a simultaneous pancreas-kidney procedure performed in 1966 by Drs Richard Lillehei and William Kelly,[1] unfortunately complicated by an early and fatal pulmonary embolism. Subsequent efforts suffered high rates of graft rejection until the introduction of cyclosporine in 1983 and thymoglobulin in 1999.[2] In the past 30 years, more than 31,000 pancreas transplant procedures have been performed in the United States with progressive improvement in surgical technique, immune suppression, and outcomes. Pancreas transplantation is currently the only curative treatment for complicated insulin-dependent diabetes, providing

Disclosures: The authors have nothing to disclose.
[a] Department of Surgery, Duke University School of Medicine, DUMC Box 3443, Room M114, Yellow Zone, Duke South, Durham, NC 27710, USA; [b] Department of Surgery, Division of Abdominal Transplant Surgery, Duke University School of Medicine, DUMC Box 3443, Room M114, Yellow Zone, Duke South, Durham, NC 27710, USA; [c] Department of Surgery, Division of Abdominal Transplant Surgery, Duke University School of Medicine, 330 Trent Drive Room 217, DUMC Box 3512, Durham, NC 27710, USA
* Corresponding author.
E-mail address: Kadiyala.Ravindra@duke.edu

Surg Clin N Am 99 (2019) 87–101
https://doi.org/10.1016/j.suc.2018.09.007
0039-6109/19/© 2018 Elsevier Inc. All rights reserved.

durable insulin independence, preventing worsening of diabetic complications, and improving quality of life.

However, the number of pancreas transplants in the United States has been steadily decreasing for the past 10 years, although recently there have been signs of recovery (**Fig. 1**). Meanwhile, outcomes for pancreas transplantation have improved: the 3-year survival after simultaneous pancreas-kidney transplantation (SPK) in 1999 to 2003 was 90.9%, compared with 94.3% for transplants performed from 2009 to 2013[3] — and the prevalence of diabetes continues to increase.[4] Decreasing transplant volumes have prompted a change in policy reducing the number of pancreas transplants required for fellow certification from 15 to 10.

TYPES OF TRANSPLANTATION

SPK is the most common type of pancreas transplant, accounting for 79% of procedures in the United States in 2016. Both organs are procured from a single deceased organ donor. A combined kidney and pancreas transplant is frequently recommended for patients with severe diabetes and chronic kidney disease.

Pancreas-after-kidney (PAK) transplantation is offered to diabetic patients who have had a kidney transplant. We plan for a PAK sequence in patients who have a viable living kidney donor identified, because the waiting time for a pancreas alone is much shorter than for a kidney-pancreas.

Pancreas transplant alone (PTA) is offered to candidates with frequent, acute, and potentially life-threatening complications of diabetes such as ketoacidosis, hypoglycemia unawareness, and incapacitating problems with insulin therapy. For this patient group, pancreas transplant can be lifesaving, but must be weighed against the risks of lifelong immunosuppression. These patients must also have stable renal function to tolerate potential calcineurin nephrotoxicity.

Living donor segmental pancreas grafts have been described,[5] with or without concurrent living donor kidney transplantation, but are not common. Although theoretically providing a better quality organ, this procedure has a high rate of donor complications, including development of pancreatic pseudocyst, pancreatic leak or fistula, requirement for splenectomy, and new-onset diabetes.

Islet cell transplantation is an appealing alternative to whole pancreas transplantation because it does not require major abdominal surgery in the recipient. However, it is not as efficacious and does still require immunosuppression. The procured pancreas is processed via variations of the Edmonton protocol[6] to isolate beta cells, which are then infused into the recipient portal vein or under the kidney capsule.

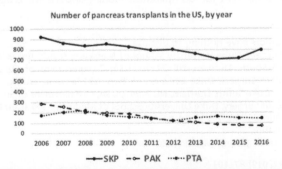

Number of pancreas transplants in the US, by year

Fig. 1. Temporal trends in pancreas transplantation in the United States 2006 to 2016. PAK, pancreas after kidney; PTA, pancreas transplant alone; SPK, simultaneous pancreas-kidney.

Multiple donors are frequently required to achieve the necessary quantity of islets. Islet cell transplantation is still considered an experimental procedure.

Listing Criteria

Although type 1 diabetes used to be a necessary criterion for pancreas transplantation candidacy, an increasing proportion of pancreas transplants are now being performed for type 2 diabetes (7.4% in 2016). A small number of pancreas transplants are also performed for chronic pancreatitis (see section on islet cell transplantation) and malignancy requiring pancreatectomy.

Patients are listed for pancreas transplant after meeting the following the United Network for Organ Sharing (UNOS) criteria:

1. Insulin therapy and absolute deficiency of endogenous insulin demonstrated by a C-peptide of less than 2 ng/mL, or
2. Insulin therapy and a C-peptide of greater than 2 ng/mL and a body mass index (BMI) of less than 28.

RECIPIENT SELECTION AND SCREENING

In addition to the UNOS criteria, patients are selected on the basis of age, BMI, and renal function. Patient and graft survival is poor in patients greater than 60 years of age, and reduced in those 50 to 59 years of age.[7] It is our practice to restrict SPK candidacy to patients less than 50 years old, with careful selection of otherwise healthy candidates 50 to 59 years of age. We use a BMI cutoff of 30, because patients with a higher BMI have worse outcomes.[8] Finally, patients should meet criteria for kidney transplant alone (glomerular filtration rate of $\leq$20 mL/min or dialysis dependence) to meet criteria for SPK.

Cardiovascular evaluation is important in pancreas transplant candidates, because cardiovascular disease remains the most common cause of death after pancreas transplantation (15% of reported cause of death). We routinely perform cardiac stress testing to identify modifiable risk factors, and proceed to cardiac catheterization if the stress test is positive.

Candidates also undergo noncontrast computed tomography scanning of the abdomen and pelvis to evaluate the caliber, position, and extent of calcification of the iliac vessels to be used for anastomosis, because peripheral vascular disease is common in this patient population. Finally, all candidates undergo the standard pretransplant psychosocial evaluation intended to evaluate social support and barriers to compliance with posttransplant care. Despite careful patient selection, wait-list mortality for SPK has been reported at 6.6% at 1 year and 54% at 5 years.[9]

DONOR SELECTION

The ideal pancreas donor is, as with most other solid organ transplants, a young healthy heart-beating donor aged 12 to 45, weighing at least 30 kg, and with a normal BMI. Donors less than 5 years old are rarely used owing to the small caliber of pancreatic vessels, which may predispose the graft to thrombosis. Donors with a BMI of greater than 30 are not routinely used for whole pancreas transplant owing to concern for fatty infiltration and a higher risk of graft pancreatitis. These donors may be good candidates for islet donation owing to higher glandular weight and islet yield.[3] Donors greater than 50 years of age have a higher risk of atherosclerosis and islet depletion and are also rarely used.

Donation after cardiac death donors are not frequently used for pancreas transplants, but may have some advantages: compared with brain-dead donors, donation after cardiac death donors are less likely to experience hyperglycemia and to release proinflammatory cytokines, which may contribute to better pancreas allograft viability.[10] The Pancreas Donor Risk Index has been developed to identify factors with an increased risk of allograft failure, but is not yet widely used.[11]

SURGICAL TECHNIQUE: PROCUREMENT
Warm Phase Dissection

The right colon, transverse colon, and base of the small bowel are mobilized to expose the aorta and inferior vena cava mesentery (Cattel-Braasch maneuver). A Kocher maneuver then delivers the duodenum and head of the pancreas. The aorta and inferior and superior mesenteric veins (IMV/SMV) are dissected and isolated for cannulation in a standard manner. The superior mesenteric artery (SMA) is dissected next and looped taking care to identify an accessory or replaced right hepatic artery arising from the SMA. The proper hepatic artery is dissected into the hilum and the gastroduodenal and splenic branches are identified and looped for division in the cold phase.

The gastrocolic ligament is divided between ties or with Ligasure or Harmonic from left to right, starting near the pylorus. The right gastroepiploic artery and vein are dissected, ligated, and divided. The short gastric vessels are divided, and the pancreas freed of its flimsy anterior attachments to the stomach. The pancreas is now well-exposed and is carefully examined for factors affecting graft quality such as fat deposition (fatty-appearing, bulky gland), atrophy, fibrosis (firm texture), or masses.

The pancreas graft is usually retrieved with the spleen to prevent injury to the distal pancreas during handling. Splenic attachments to the diaphragm and left colon flexure are taken down and the spleen is mobilized. Care should be taken to prevent injury to the pancreatic tail, which may be encountered during posterior splenic mobilization. The dissection is continued posteriorly using the spleen as a handle, and the pancreas is mobilized from the retroperitoneum to the level of the IMV, preserving the IMV for cannulation.

Before cross-clamping, a mixture of antimicrobials and antifungals is delivered into the stomach and duodenum through nasogastric tube. The jejunum is divided with a GIA stapler close to duodenojenunal junction. At this stage, the warm phase pancreas dissection is complete.

Cold Phase Dissection

Before cannulation, systemic heparinization is done with intravenous heparin 300 U/kg. The aorta and IMV are cannulated 3 minutes after heparinization. Aortic cross-clamping, organ flush, and inferior vena cava venting in chest or abdomen are done in sequence and the organs perfused with 3 to 4 L of cold perfusate through the aorta and 2 L through the portal vein. The most commonly used solutions are University of Wisconsin solution or histidine–tryptophan–ketoglutarate. The liver graft is procured first, followed by the pancreas. The liver and pancreas may also be procured together and separated on the back table.

The anterior wall of the aorta is divided in the midline from its bifurcation until the SMA. The SMA is divided at its insertion or procured on a single patch with the celiac artery. If the right hepatic artery arises from the SMA close to its origin, the SMA is divided beyond the takeoff of right hepatic. In rare cases, the right hepatic artery courses through the pancreas parenchyma and must be dissected out to go with the liver graft, in which case a usable pancreas graft cannot be procured. The dorsal pancreatic artery usually arises from the splenic artery to provide blood supply to the pancreatic tail. When the dorsal pancreatic artery arises from the common hepatic artery or the celiac trunk, it is vulnerable to unintentional injury during back-table dissection.[12,13] This process may compromise blood supply to the pancreatic tail.

The gastroduodenal artery is tied and divided. The splenic artery is divided to leave sufficient length with the pancreas graft for back-table reconstruction. The portal vein is divided next, about 1 cm above the duodenum. The stomach is stapled proximal to the pylorus. The small bowel mesentery containing the infrapancreatic SMA and SMV is divided away from the inferior border of pancreas with a vascular stapler, taking care to preserve the inferior pancreaticoduodenal arteries. Alternatively, the SMA and SMV can be ligated and divided individually. The remaining attachments are divided and the pancreas graft is removed.

Back Table

The spleen is removed carefully to avoid parenchymal injury to the pancreas, and peripancreatic tissue and fat are cleared. The IMV is ligated. The duodenal segment is shortened by stapling the proximal end just distal to the pylorus, taking care to preserve pancreatic duct drainage. Both staple lines at the proximal and distal duodenal ends are inverted with running Prolene sutures. The mesenteric staple line is also overrun. Vascular reconstruction may now be performed with the donor iliac artery bifurcation used as a Y-graft to provide single inflow to the splenic artery and SMA (**Figs. 2** and **3**). The venous outflow should not be extended with a graft owing to a higher risk of venous thrombosis. On the back table, completeness of the pancreatic vascular arcade may be assessed using gentle fluid flush or with an angiogram.

SURGICAL TECHNIQUE: PRESERVATION

The pancreas graft is stored in UW or histidine–tryptophan–ketoglutarate solution, packed, and transported in an ice-lined box to the recipient hospital. Cold ischemic time is optimally kept less than 12 hours. Although pulsatile preservation is used with success in kidneys, it is not yet commonplace for pancreas grafts. Studies of cold perfusion have largely been done in the context of islet cell transplantations, and have not as of yet demonstrated an optimal technique or clear benefit.[12–15]

SURGICAL TECHNIQUE: IMPLANTATION, VASCULAR

The recipient incision may be placed in the right iliac fossa, transversely, or in the midline depending on anticipated graft placement. The ascending colon and root of

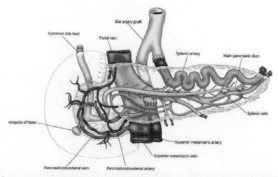

Fig. 2. Diagram of prepared pancreas allograft with donor iliac artery Y-graft arterial reconstruction. (*Illustrated by* Megan Llewellyn, MSMI; copyright Duke University; with permission under a CC BY-ND 4.0 license [Creative Commons Attribution-NoDerivatives 4.0 International License].)

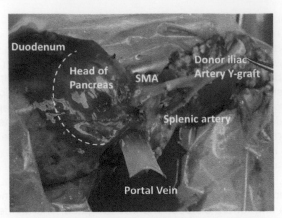

Fig. 3. Back-table preparation of pancreas allograft with donor iliac artery Y-graft. SMA, superior mesenteric artery.

the small bowel mesentery are mobilized to expose the right common iliac artery and inferior vena cava. When transplanted simultaneously with a kidney, the pancreas is implanted first to minimize ischemic time.

Several procedural variations exist for pancreas vascular and enteric anastomoses. At our center, we commonly place the pancreas in the right pelvis with systemic venous outflow to the common or external iliac vein, and perform the arterial anastomosis to the common or external iliac artery (**Figs. 4** and **5**).

The pancreas may also be placed on the small bowel mesentery, with arterial inflow from the iliac artery or aorta and venous outflow to the portal vein or SMV (**Fig. 6**). Although systemic drainage is technically easier, the recipient runs the risk of hyperinsulinemia. Portal drainage is theoretically more physiologic, allowing pancreatic endocrine secretions first-pass metabolism through the liver. Portal venous drainage, however, has not demonstrated an advantage over systemic drainage in terms of graft

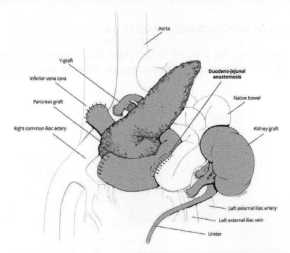

Fig. 4. Diagram of pancreas allograft in situ: systemic venous drainage via inferior vena cava and enteric exocrine drainage via duodenojejunostomy. Kidney allograft in left iliac fossa. (*Illustrated by* Megan Llewellyn, MSMI; copyright Duke University; with permission under a CC BY-ND 4.0 license [Creative Commons Attribution-NoDerivatives 4.0 International License].)

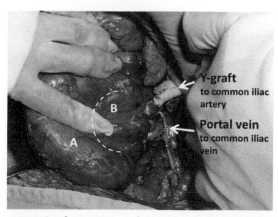

Fig. 5. Vascular anastomosis of pancreas graft to right common iliac artery and vein, using donor iliac artery Y-graft for arterial reconstruction. (A) Allograft duodenum. (B) Allograft pancreatic head.

function or long-term survival.[14–16] According to a 2011 International Pancreas Transplant Registry report,[17] 82% of SPK and 90% of PTA worldwide are performed with systemic venous drainage.

SURGICAL TECHNIQUE: IMPLANTATION, EXOCRINE

The original described technique of pancreas graft exocrine drainage was to the bladder. Although fraught with complications (metabolic acidosis, cystitis, urinary tract infections, and reflux pancreatitis from urinary retention, among others), bladder drainage allowed monitoring of urinary amylase for earlier diagnosis of graft rejection. This factor became less important as immunosuppression improved. Enteric drainage was first performed in 1981 and became widely used in the late 1990s, when thymoglobulin induction of immunosuppression was standardized.[2]

Depending on the placement of the organ, enteric drainage is performed with either a duodenojejunostomy or a Roux-en-Y limb. According to UNOS data from 2006 to 2016, 8.4% of pancreas were performed with bladder drainage, 18.5% with enteric drainage using a Roux limb, and 66.4% with enteric drainage without a Roux limb. Patient and graft survival are similar for both strategies,[18] although bladder-drained grafts may have to be revised to enteric drainage owing to complications. At our center, we perform enteric drainage exclusively (**Fig. 7**).

Duodenoduodenostomy is a recently developed exocrine drainage technique intended to facilitate access to the transplanted pancreas for endoscopic biopsy and intervention. The donor duodenum is anastomosed side-to-side to D2/D3 of the recipient duodenum, the graft placed in a right-sided retrocolic position, and vascular anastomoses made to the right common iliac and lower inferior vena cava (see **Fig. 6**). This technique has not yet been shown to improve clinical outcomes.[19–21]

IMMUNOSUPPRESSION

Owing to a higher rate of rejection and greater difficulty in diagnosis, higher levels of immune suppression are used for pancreas transplants compared with kidney transplant alone. T-cell–depleting agents are used routinely for pancreas recipients, but only selectively for kidney recipients who are higher risk. Randomized trials have

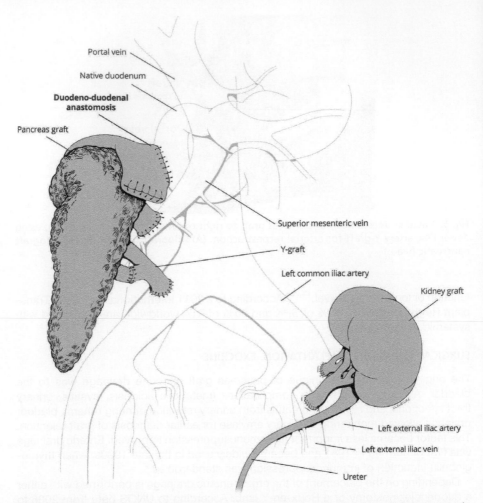

Portal vein

Native duodenum

Duodeno-duodenal anastomosis

Pancreas graft

Superior mesenteric vein

Y-graft

Left common iliac artery

Kidney graft

Left external iliac artery

Left external iliac vein

Ureter

Fig. 6. Diagram of pancreas allograft in situ: portal venous drainage via superior mesenteric vein and enteric exocrine drainage via duodenoduodenostomy. Kidney allograft in left iliac fossa. (*Illustrated by* Megan Llewellyn, MSMI; copyright Duke University; with permission under a CC BY-ND 4.0 license [Creative Commons Attribution-NoDerivatives 4.0 International License].)

securely demonstrated the superiority of antithymocyte globulin (ATG) induction over azathioprine for improving graft and patient survival.[22] Other induction regimens are under investigation including basiliximab, alemtuzumab, and rabbit ATG,[23–26] although none are yet demonstrably superior to ATG.

Maintenance regimens typically consist of a calcineurin inhibitor, mycophenolate, and a low-dose corticosteroid. Tacrolimus is used most frequently and may have a pancreas graft survival advantage when compared with cyclosporine.[27] Mycophenolate mofetil is the most commonly used antimetabolite for maintenance therapy. Compared with azathioprine, mycophenolate mofetil decreases the incidence and severity of acute cellular rejection and improves graft survival.[28] Some centers use a steroid-free regimen or withdraw prednisone after some period of stability, although there is not yet sufficient evidence for the effect of this strategy on long-term pancreas outcomes.[29] At our center, all pancreas transplant recipients receive ATG induction

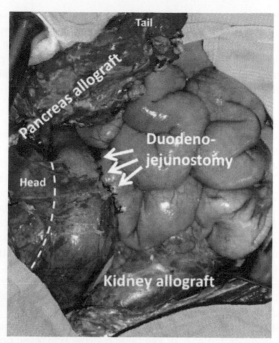

Fig. 7. Simultaneous pancreas and kidney allografts in situ; enteric exocrine drainage via duodenojejunostomy.

and maintenance with prednisone, mycophenolate mofetil, and a calcineurin inhibitor; tacrolimus levels are titrated to 10 ng/mL for the first 6 months after transplantation.

The use of mammalian target of rapamycin inhibitors (sirolimus, everolimus, rapamycin) has been decreasing to only 10% of pancreas patients transplanted in recent years.[30] This finding is likely due to consideration of the nephrotoxic and diabetogenic side effects of these drugs without a clear graft survival advantage. Mammalian target of rapamycin inhibitors remain a valuable second-line maintenance treatment.

COMPLICATIONS
Early Complications

Early graft loss is most frequently owing to graft thrombosis, which complicates 5% to 10% of pancreas transplants. Contributing causes include technical error, hypoperfusion, pancreatitis, atherosclerosis, and torsion of the vascular pedicle. Graft thrombosis is diagnosed by rapid elevation in serum glucose and amylase and is treated by urgent pancreatectomy.

Early postoperative hemorrhage is typically due to small vessel bleeding and may be avoided by careful back-table preparation. Transplant pancreatitis is a rare complication (3%), thought to be due to reperfusion injury, aggressive resuscitation, and poor tissue handling. Graft pancreatitis is difficult to diagnose and to distinguish from acute rejection, and patients should be treated for rejection until proven otherwise. Pancreatitis rarely contributes to graft failure (<1%).

Pancreatic Anastomotic Leak

Anastomotic leak is a rare but serious complication, contributing to 4% of graft failures. The diagnosis is suggested by peritonitis, fever, leukocytosis, and confirmed by computed tomography scanning with oral contrast (for enteric-drained grafts). Depending on the source of the leak, it may be reasonable to attempt debridement and surgical repair, and treatment with somatostatin to decrease the volume of pancreatic secretions.[31] If the leak is at the duodenal anastomosis, pancreatectomy is preferred because the enteric anastomosis is likely contaminated with active pancreatic enzymes and unlikely to heal.

Graft Rejection

Pancreas transplants are particularly susceptible to graft rejection, with an incidence of 15% to 21% at 1 year and 27% to 30% at 5 years.[32,33] Compare this finding with kidney transplantation alone, where rejection incidence is approximately 10% at 1 year and 20% at 5 years.[34] In SPKs, pancreas rejection has a concordance of 60% with kidney graft rejection and lags in severity.[35] Rejection of the pancreas allograft alone is difficult to diagnose, and is suggested by clinical findings of fever and graft tenderness. Multiple serum markers are used to monitor graft function including glucose, amylase, lipase, and C-peptide levels. Of these, lipase is the most specific.[36]

If rejection is suspected, patients should undergo a graft ultrasound examination with Doppler to rule out vascular complication or peripancreatic fluid collection, possibly followed by computed tomography scanning and biopsy. Biopsy of the pancreas allograft has a 2.8% complication rate and is frequently (12%) nondiagnostic owing to technical challenge and sampling error. Before treatment, graft function is confirmed by measuring fasting glucose, C-peptide, and hemoglobin A1c. Elevated fasting glucose or hemoglobin A1c, or low fasting C-peptide level, portend poor graft survival. In this case, treatment of graft rejection may not be worth the risk.[36]

The treatment for acute cellular rejection of the pancreas allograft is typically high dose steroids with or without thymoglobulin. In the UNOS dataset, 4.5% of graft losses are attributed to acute rejection.

Infections

Pancreas transplant recipients are at risk for the standard set of posttransplant viral, bacterial, and fungal infections. Patients receiving thymoglobulin induction are at higher risk of cytomegalovirus viremia. SPK and PAK recipients are also at risk for BK virus.

OUTCOMES

Pancreas transplant is associated with an all-cause mortality rate of 4% at 1 year and 9% at 5 years. The single most common cause of death is cardiovascular. SPK recipients have better long-term survival than deceased-donor kidney-alone transplant recipients (72% vs 55% at 8 years), and comparable survival to living-donor kidney recipients (72% at 8 years).[37] Patients receiving a pancreas after kidney transplants have an early increase in mortality, but trend toward better long-term survival when compared with patients receiving a kidney alone.[38,39] PAK patients also have better long-term kidney graft function than patients with a kidney alone.[40]

Graft survival defined as insulin independence and a normal hemoglobin A1c is reported at 86% at 1 year and 54% at 10 years for SPK recipients.[41] PAK and PTA graft survival is lower, perhaps because serum creatinine is not available as a marker of graft rejection. Graft outcomes are inversely related to recipient age, donor age, BMI, the Donor Risk Index, and the burden of cardiovascular disease.[11] The most common causes of graft loss are thrombosis (31%), chronic rejection (21%), and acute rejection (15%).

OUTCOMES: METABOLIC

Successful pancreas transplantation results in enduring independence from insulin therapy, reported out to 15 years.[42] Patients have improvement in glucose metabolism and counterregulatory responses to insulin-induced hypoglycemia,[43] as well as improvements in serum lipids and endothelial function.[44–46] Hypoglycemia is uncommon after pancreas transplantation and is usually mild.[47]

Pancreas transplantation leads to many improvements in microvascular complications of chronic diabetes, including the following.

- Nephropathy: prevention and improvement of existing disease.[48]
- Neuropathy: stabilization and improvement of motor and sensory nerve conduction,[49–54] although no evidence for improvement of gastric emptying.
- Retinopathy: conflicting evidence with some reports of stabilization and improvement.[55–57] Cataracts may worsen owing to treatment with calcineurin inhibitors and steroids.[58]

There are not yet adequate data to evaluate the effect of pancreas transplant on chronic macrovascular complications of diabetes. Some studied intermediaries include the following.

- Regression of coronary atherosclerosis in 38% of SPK recipients with working grafts.[59]
- Increased[60] or decreased[61] carotid intimal thickness after SPK, insufficient evidence about CVA (cardiovascular accident) outcomes.
- No improvement in trajectory of peripheral vascular disease[62,63]

OUTCOMES: ISLETS

Islet cell transplant outcomes have improved from insulin independence of 27% at 3 years (1999–2002) to 44% (2007–2010).[64] These rates are still inferior to whole organ pancreas transplant, with recently reported insulin independence rates of 69% to 85% at 3 years for PTA.[65] No evidence adequately describes the effect of islet cell transplant on the vascular complications of diabetes. There is insufficient evidence to determine whether the benefits of islet cell transplant outweigh the risks of long-term immunosuppression.

Islet cell autotransplantation is an emerging method of preserving pancreatic endocrine function after total pancreatectomy for chronic pancreatitis. Insulin independence rates vary with islet yield and are reported to be as high as 72% at 3 years.[66] This procedure does not require immunosuppression.

ACKNOWLEDGMENTS

The authors would like to thank Megan Llewelyn for the included illustrations.

REFERENCES

1. Kelly WD, Lillehei RC, Merkel FK, et al. Allotransplantation of the pancreas and duodenum along with the kidney in diabetic nephropathy. Surgery 1967;61(6): 827–37.
2. Sutherland DE, Gruessner RW, Dunn DL, et al. Lessons learned from more than 1,000 pancreas transplants at a single institution. Ann Surg 2001;233(4):463–501.
3. Stratta RJ, Gruessner AC, Odorico JS, et al. Pancreas transplantation: an alarming crisis in confidence. Am J Transplant 2016;16(9):2556–62.

4. Temporal trends in recording of diabetes on death certificates | diabetes care. Available at: http://care.diabetesjournals.org/content/34/7/1529. Accessed April 19, 2018.
5. Sutherland DE, Gruessner R, Dunn D, et al. Pancreas transplants from living-related donors. Transplant Proc 1994;26(2):443–5.
6. Shapiro AMJ, Ricordi C, Hering BJ, et al. International trial of the Edmonton protocol for islet transplantation. N Engl J Med 2006;355(13):1318–30.
7. Siskind E, Maloney C, Akerman M, et al. An analysis of pancreas transplantation outcomes based on age groupings–an update of the UNOS database. Clin Transplant 2014;28(9):990–4.
8. Sampaio MS, Reddy PN, Kuo H-T, et al. Obesity was associated with inferior outcomes in simultaneous pancreas kidney transplant. Transplantation 2010;89(9): 1117–25.
9. Gruessner RWG, Sutherland DER, Gruessner AC. Mortality assessment for pancreas transplants. Am J Transplant 2004;4(12):2018–26.
10. Ridgway D, Manas D, Shaw J, et al. Preservation of the donor pancreas for whole pancreas and islet transplantation. Clin Transplant 2010;24(1):1–19.
11. Axelrod DA, Sung RS, Meyer KH, et al. Systematic evaluation of pancreas allograft quality, outcomes and geographic variation in utilization. Am J Transplant 2010;10(4):837–45.
12. Baranski AG, Lam H-D, Braat AE, et al. The dorsal pancreatic artery in pancreas procurement and transplantation: anatomical considerations and potential implications. Clin Transplant 2016;30(10):1360–4.
13. Okahara M, Mori H, Kiyosue H, et al. Arterial supply to the pancreas; variations and cross-sectional anatomy. Abdom Imaging 2010;35(2):134–42.
14. Oliver JB, Beidas A-K, Bongu A, et al. A comparison of long-term outcomes of portal versus systemic venous drainage in pancreatic transplantation: a systematic review and meta-analysis. Clin Transplant 2015;29(10):882–92.
15. Bazerbachi F, Selzner M, Marquez MA, et al. Portal venous versus systemic venous drainage of pancreas grafts: impact on long-term results. Am J Transplant 2012;12(1):226–32.
16. Havrdova T, Boucek P, Jedinakova T, et al. Portal versus systemic venous drainage of the pancreatic graft: the effect on glucose metabolism in pancreas and kidney transplant recipients. Transplant Proc 2014;46(6):1910–2.
17. Gruessner AC, Gruessner RWG. Pancreas transplantation of US and non-US cases from 2005 to 2014 as reported to the United Network for Organ Sharing (UNOS) and the International Pancreas Transplant Registry (IPTR). Rev Diabet Stud 2016;13(1):35–58.
18. Mai ML, Ahsan N, Gonwa T. The long-term management of pancreas transplantation. Transplantation 2006;82(8):991–1003.
19. Lindahl JP, Horneland R, Nordheim E, et al. Outcomes in pancreas transplantation with exocrine drainage through a duodenoduodenostomy versus duodenojejunostomy. Am J Transplant 2018;18(1):154–62.
20. Walter M, Jazra M, Kykalos S, et al. 125 Cases of duodenoduodenostomy in pancreas transplantation: a single-centre experience of an alternative enteric drainage. Transpl Int 2014;27(8):805–15.
21. Horneland R, Paulsen V, Lindahl JP, et al. Pancreas transplantation with enteroanastomosis to native duodenum poses technical challenges–but offers improved endoscopic access for scheduled biopsies and therapeutic interventions. Am J Transplant 2015;15(1):242–50.

22. Burke GW, Kaufman DB, Millis JM, et al. Prospective, randomized trial of the effect of antibody induction in simultaneous pancreas and kidney transplantation: three-year results. Transplantation 2004;77(8):1269–75.

23. Bazerbachi F, Selzner M, Boehnert MU, et al. Thymoglobulin versus basiliximab induction therapy for simultaneous kidney-pancreas transplantation: impact on rejection, graft function, and long-term outcome. Transplantation 2011;92(9): 1039–43.

24. Fernández-Burgos I, Montiel Casado MC, Pérez-Daga JA, et al. Induction therapy in simultaneous pancreas-kidney transplantation: thymoglobulin versus basiliximab. Transplant Proc 2015;47(1):120–2.

25. Farney AC, Doares W, Rogers J, et al. A randomized trial of alemtuzumab versus antithymocyte globulin induction in renal and pancreas transplantation. Transplantation 2009;88(6):810–9.

26. Stratta RJ, Rogers J, Orlando G, et al. 5-year results of a prospective, randomized, single-center study of alemtuzumab compared with rabbit antithymocyte globulin induction in simultaneous kidney-pancreas transplantation. Transplant Proc 2014;46(6):1928–31.

27. Saudek F, Malaise J, Boucek P, et al, Euro-SPK Study Group. Efficacy and safety of tacrolimus compared with cyclosporin microemulsion in primary SPK transplantation: 3-year results of the Euro-SPK 001 trial. Nephrol Dial Transplant 2005;20(Suppl 2):ii3–10, ii62.

28. Merion RM, Henry ML, Melzer JS, et al. Randomized, prospective trial of mycophenolate mofetil versus azathioprine for prevention of acute renal allograft rejection after simultaneous kidney-pancreas transplantation. Transplantation 2000; 70(1):105–11.

29. Montero N, Webster AC, Royuela A, et al. Steroid avoidance or withdrawal for pancreas and pancreas with kidney transplant recipients. Cochrane Database Syst Rev 2014;(9):CD007669.

30. Kandaswamy R, Stock PG, Gustafson SK, et al. OPTN/SRTR 2015 annual data report: pancreas. Am J Transplant 2017;17(S1):117–73.

31. Al-Adra D, McGilvray I, Goldaracena N, et al. Preserving the pancreas graft: outcomes of surgical repair of duodenal leaks in enterically drained pancreas allografts. Transplant Direct 2017;3(7):e179.

32. Dong M, Parsaik AK, Kremers W, et al. Acute pancreas allograft rejection is associated with increased risk of graft failure in pancreas transplantation. Am J Transplant 2013;13(4):1019–25.

33. Niederhaus SV, Leverson GE, Lorentzen DF, et al. Acute cellular and antibody-mediated rejection of the pancreas allograft: incidence, risk factors and outcomes. Am J Transplant 2013;13(11):2945–55.

34. Matas AJ, Smith JM, Skeans MA, et al. OPTN/SRTR 2012 annual data report: kidney. Am J Transplant 2014;14(Suppl 1):11–44.

35. Shapiro R, Jordan ML, Scantlebury VP, et al. Renal allograft rejection with normal renal function in simultaneous kidney/pancreas recipients: does dissynchronous rejection really exist? Transplantation 2000;69(3):440–1.

36. Redfield RR, Kaufman DB, Odorico JS. Diagnosis and treatment of pancreas rejection. Curr Transplant Rep 2015;2(2):169–75.

37. Reddy KS, Stablein D, Taranto S, et al. Long-term survival following simultaneous kidney-pancreas transplantation versus kidney transplantation alone in patients with type 1 diabetes mellitus and renal failure. Am J Kidney Dis 2003;41(2): 464–70.

38. Venstrom JM, McBride MA, Rother KI, et al. Survival after pancreas transplantation in patients with diabetes and preserved kidney function. JAMA 2003;290(21): 2817–23.

39. Sampaio MS, Poommipanit N, Cho YW, et al. Transplantation with pancreas after living donor kidney vs. living donor kidney alone in type 1 diabetes mellitus recipients. Clin Transplant 2010;24(6):812–20.

40. Francois K, Martin F, Sutherland David ER, et al. Pancreas after living donor kidney transplants in diabetic patients: impact on long-term kidney graft function. Clin Transplant 2009;23(4):437–46.

41. Gruessner AC. 2011 update on pancreas transplantation: comprehensive trend analysis of 25,000 cases followed up over the course of twenty-four years at the International Pancreas Transplant Registry (IPTR). Rev Diabet Stud 2011; 8(1):6–16.

42. Robertson RP, Sutherland DE, Lanz KJ. Normoglycemia and preserved insulin secretory reserve in diabetic patients 10-18 years after pancreas transplantation. Diabetes 1999;48(9):1737–40.

43. Robertson RP, Sutherland DE, Kendall DM, et al. Metabolic characterization of long-term successful pancreas transplants in type I diabetes. J Investig Med 1996;44(9):549–55.

44. Larsen JL, Stratta RJ, Ozaki CF, et al. Lipid status after pancreas-kidney transplantation. Diabetes Care 1992;15(1):35–42.

45. La Rocca E, Secchi A, Parlavecchia M, et al. Lipid metabolism after successful kidney and pancreatic transplantation. Transplant Proc 1991;23(1 Pt 2):1672–3.

46. Fiorina P, La Rocca E, Venturini M, et al. Effects of kidney-pancreas transplantation on atherosclerotic risk factors and endothelial function in patients with uremia and type 1 diabetes. Diabetes 2001;50(3):496–501.

47. Shen J, Gaglia J. Hypoglycemia following pancreas transplantation. Curr Diab Rep 2008;8(4):317–23.

48. Fioretto P, Steffes MW, Sutherland DE, et al. Reversal of lesions of diabetic nephropathy after pancreas transplantation. N Engl J Med 1998;339(2):69–75.

49. Allen RD, Al-Harbi IS, Morris JG, et al. Diabetic neuropathy after pancreas transplantation: determinants of recovery. Transplantation 1997;63(6):830–8.

50. Aridge D, Reese J, Niehoff M, et al. Effect of successful renal and segmental pancreatic transplantation on peripheral and autonomic neuropathy. Transplant Proc 1991;23(1 Pt 2):1670–1.

51. Gaber AO, Cardoso S, Pearson S, et al. Improvement in autonomic function following combined pancreas-kidney transplantation. Transplant Proc 1991; 23(1 Pt 2):1660–2.

52. Navarro X, Kennedy WR, Loewenson RB, et al. Influence of pancreas transplantation on cardiorespiratory reflexes, nerve conduction, and mortality in diabetes mellitus. Diabetes 1990;39(7):802–6.

53. Navarro X, Sutherland DE, Kennedy WR. Long-term effects of pancreatic transplantation on diabetic neuropathy. Ann Neurol 1997;42(5):727–36.

54. Secchi A, Martinenghi S, Galardi G, et al. Effects of pancreatic transplantation on diabetic polyneuropathy. Transplant Proc 1991;23(1 Pt 2):1658–9.

55. Pearce IA, Ilango B, Sells RA, et al. Stabilisation of diabetic retinopathy following simultaneous pancreas and kidney transplant. Br J Ophthalmol 2000;84(7): 736–40.

56. Königsrainer A, Miller K, Steurer W, et al. Does pancreas transplantation influence the course of diabetic retinopathy? Diabetologia 1991;34(Suppl 1):S86–8.

57. Ramsay RC, Goetz FC, Sutherland DE, et al. Progression of diabetic retinopathy after pancreas transplantation for insulin-dependent diabetes mellitus. N Engl J Med 1988;318(4):208–14.
58. Pai RP, Mitchell P, Chow VC, et al. Posttransplant cataract: lessons from kidney-pancreas transplantation. Transplantation 2000;69(6):1108–14.
59. Jukema JW, Smets YFC, van der Pijl JW, et al. Impact of simultaneous pancreas and kidney transplantation on progression of coronary atherosclerosis in patients with end-stage renal failure due to type 1 diabetes. Diabetes Care 2002;25(5): 906–11.
60. Nankivell BJ, Lau SG, Chapman JR, et al. Progression of macrovascular disease after transplantation. Transplantation 2000;69(4):574–81.
61. Larsen JL, Colling CW, Ratanasuwan T, et al. Pancreas transplantation improves vascular disease in patients with type 1 diabetes. Diabetes Care 2004;27(7): 1706–11.
62. Bruce DS, Newell KA, Josephson MA, et al. Long-term outcome of kidney-pancreas transplant recipients with good graft function at one year. Transplantation 1996;62(4):451–6.
63. Long-term effects of pancreatic transplant function in patients with advanced juvenile-onset diabetes | Diabetes Care. Available at: http://care.diabetesjournals.org/content/1/1/1. Accessed May 29, 2018.
64. Barton FB, Rickels MR, Alejandro R, et al. Improvement in outcomes of clinical islet transplantation: 1999–2010. Diabetes Care 2012;35(7):1436–45.
65. Gruessner RWG, Gruessner AC. Pancreas transplant alone: a procedure coming of age. Diabetes Care 2013;36(8):2440–7.
66. Sutherland DER, Radosevich DM, Bellin MD, et al. Total pancreatectomy and islet autotransplantation for chronic pancreatitis. J Am Coll Surg 2012;214(4):409–24 [discussion: 424–6].

Small Bowel Transplantation

Samuel Kesseli, MD[a], Debra Sudan, MD[b],*

KEYWORDS

- Small bowel transplantation • Intestinal transplantation • Short bowel syndrome
- Intestinal failure

KEY POINTS

- The primary therapy for intestinal failure is total parenteral nutrition, and small bowel transplantation is reserved generally for patients who develop life-threatening complications related to total parenteral nutrition administration.
- Given that small bowel transplantation is an infrequently performed procedure, individual centers have inadequate case volume to identify optimal surgical techniques and timing. Multicenter studies are crucial to advance knowledge in this field.
- Intestine allografts are more immunogenic than other solid organ allografts and, therefore, patients experience more acute rejection episodes, require higher levels/doses of immunosuppressive medications, and have a higher incidence of infectious complications related to immunosuppression than recipients of other solid organ allografts.
- The significance of antibody development (especially donor-specific antibody) in intestine transplant candidates or recipients and antibody-mediated rejection is less well defined than in kidney and heart transplantation and is the target of current investigations in the field.

INTRODUCTION: NATURE OF THE PROBLEM AND INDICATIONS

Intestinal failure (IF) is defined clinically as any cause of gastrointestinal (GI) dysfunction that results in the inability to meet nutritional demands, necessitating either temporary or indefinite dependence on parenteral nutrition (PN).[1] Most often this occurs secondary to surgical resection, leading to short bowel syndrome, although functional disorders in motility, mucosal defects, obstruction, and fistulae may also account for IF.[2,3] Quantitatively, IF can be assessed with biomarkers of functional enterocyte mass (ie, citrulline) or energy absorption studies; however, these tests may not accurately predict a patient's PN requirement and are not available in all centers and, therefore, are of limited clinical utility.[4–6] As such, IF is frequently a clinical diagnosis made in

Disclosure Statement: The authors have nothing to disclose.
[a] Department of Surgery, Duke University Medical Center, Durham, NC, USA; [b] Division of Abdominal Transplant Surgery, Duke University Medical Center, DUMC Box 3522, Durham, NC 27710, USA
* Corresponding author.
E-mail address: Debra.sudan@duke.edu

Surg Clin N Am 99 (2019) 103–116
https://doi.org/10.1016/j.suc.2018.09.008
0039-6109/19/© 2018 Elsevier Inc. All rights reserved.
surgical.theclinics.com

patients with fluid and electrolyte abnormalities and protein-calorie malnutrition that preclude nutritional autonomy.

Regardless of the cause, the primary first-line therapy for IF remains PN. Although this approach is dependable, it comes with morbidity related to catheter-associated infections,[7] venous thrombosis,[8,9] and IF-associated liver disease (IFALD).[10] Furthermore, these patients require frequent monitoring due to electrolyte abnormalities, dehydration, and vitamin deficiencies. Overall, for patients with IF of nonmalignant etiologies, 1-year and 5-year survival rates on chronic PN have been reported from 86% to 97% and 58% to 83%, respectively. Furthermore, a recent study from Europe suggests mortality in PN-dependent patients is most often the result of the underlying disease process, and PN-associated complications account for patient death in 14% of IF patients.[11]

Given the efficacy of PN for treatment of IF, intestinal transplantation (IT) is reserved for patients who have failed PN. The definitions for failed PN therapy accepted by the Centers for Medicare & Medicaid Services are listed in **Box 1**.[12] These indications have not been updated since 2006 and do not include indications proposed in more recent literature, such as portomesenteric thrombosis, frozen abdomen, and benign or slow-growing abdominal tumors that involve the hilum of the liver.[13,14] For these patients with more recently defined indications, multivisceral transplantation with removal of affected segments of the GI tract may be the best or only life-saving therapy available.

THERAPEUTIC OPTIONS AND SURGICAL TECHNIQUE

Prior to considering IT, nontransplant surgical techniques are frequently used for autologous GI reconstruction (AGIR) to improve intestine function and decrease total PN (TPN) dependence and the associated complications. These have been thoroughly reviewed elsewhere[15] and are not the focus of this article. In cases of these AGIR surgeries not possible or not successful, IT alone or in combination with other abdominal organs may be a viable option.

Most commonly, IT is performed using the isolated small bowel graft, which accounts for 46% of transplanted grafts in the most recent series published by the

---

Box 1
Current accepted indications for intestinal transplantation per the Medicare national coverage determination

1. Recurrent catheter-associated bloodstream infection
   - Two or more line infections per year
   - A single episode of fungal infection
   - Development of septic shock or acute respiratory distress syndrome

2. IFALD
   - Characterized by elevated liver enzymes, elevated bilirubin, splenomegaly, thrombocytopenia, gastroesophageal varices, coagulopathy

3. Complications of venous thrombosis
   - Thrombosis of 2 or more major central vessels
   - Loss of venous access
   - Sepsis secondary to infected thrombi
   - Pulmonary embolism

4. Frequent episodes of dehydration where fluid losses exceed maximum infusion rates

5. Transplant performed at a center with annual volume greater than 10 per year

Intestinal Transplant Registry (ITR).[16] This graft uses the entirety of donor jejunum and ileum anastomosed to the recipient proximal jejunum. The vascular pedicle consists of the superior mesenteric artery (SMA) and superior mesenteric vein (SMV) (**Fig. 1**A), which are anastomosed directly to the infrarenal aorta and vena cava. An ileostomy is then created from the distal ileum of the allograft in most instances with or without anastomosis of the distal small bowel with native colon (see **Fig. 1**B). Many surgeons now opt to include a segment of donor colon with these grafts (not shown), because inclusion of the ileocecal valve is associated with improved quality of life, continence, and independence from PN.[16,17]

The combined liver-intestine graft (**Fig. 2**) is considered in patients with IF and concomitant IFALD. With this technique, the pancreaticoduodenal complex is preserved and the liver, inferior vena cava (IVC), pancreas, spleen, and small bowel (including duodenum) are resected from the donor en bloc with a segment of thoracic aorta, which includes the celiac axis SMA. The spleen is typically removed on the back table prior to graft implantation although some centers have reported removal after reperfusion of the graft or even transplantation of the spleen as part of the allograft. On implantation, the suprahepatic and infrahepatic IVC anastomoses are created

A   **B**

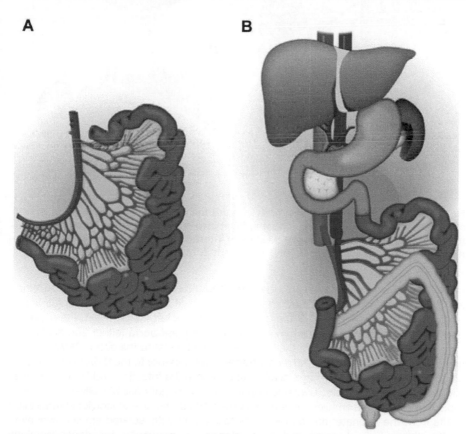

Fig. 1. The isolated small bowel graft. (*A*) The vascular pedicle consists of the SMA and SMV. (*B*) The graft is anastomosed with the recipient jejunum and terminates in an ileostomy. The graft may or may not be placed in continuity with colon. (*From* Sudan D. The current state of intestine transplantation: indications, techniques, outcomes and challenges. Am J Transplant 2014;14(9):1976–84; with permission.)

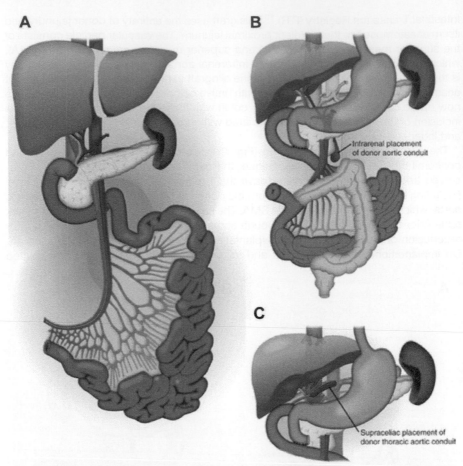

Fig. 2. The combined liver-intestinal graft includes the pancreaticoduodenal complex with or without spleen (*A*). The donor aorta may be anastomosed infrarenally (*B*) or to supraceliac aorta (*C*). (*From* Sudan D. The current state of intestine transplantation: indications, techniques, outcomes and challenges. Am J Transplant 2014;14(9):1976–84; with permission.)

(or for piggyback implantation only the suprahepatic IVC anastomosis) and the recipient portal vein is sewn to the donor portal system (if the full donor pancreas is not retained) or the recipient IVC (if the donor pancreas is left intact). Next, the proximal end of the donor aorta is anastomosed to the recipient aorta (either supraceliac or infrarenal) and the distal end of the donor aorta (just distal to the donor SMA) is oversewn. In small infants, where the renal arteries arise superior to the SMA takeoff, patch closure of the donor aorta may still allow use of both the intestine and individual renal allografts, although en bloc pediatric donor kidneys are not possible. Given that this is most common in the smallest donors, less than 10 kg, the size of individual renal allografts from the neonate may be too small to use. As with isolated small bowel allografts, the proximal small bowel is placed in continuity by donor-recipient jejunojejunal and ileocolic anastomoses.[18]

The term, *multivisceral, transplantation*, has been used by different centers to refer the liver-intestine allograft, described previously, if the recipient native foregut is removed, or by other centers to describe inclusion of additional organs, such as stomach or colon in the liver-intestine allograft. Although the role of incorporating stomach remains unclear, splenic preservation has been shown to provide a reduction in graft rejection rates but an increased risk of autoimmune hemolysis[19] and graft-versus-host disease (GVHD)[20] and, therefore, has not become standard of care.

CLINICAL OUTCOMES AND COMPLICATIONS

Currently there are approximately 30 centers in the United States that have performed IT and more than than 80 centers worldwide. North America accounts for 76% of the global case volume.[16] In the United States, the most recent regional data from the Organ Procurement and Transplantation Network demonstrate that the number of ITs has declined over the last decade from its peak in 2007 (198) to only 109 transplants performed in 2017 (**Fig. 3**). This decline may be the result of improved treatment of and prevention of IFALD through improved liver-sparing lipid emulsions and multidisciplinary IF care,[21] but, given the small volume of centers, access to care may also play a role.

Given the relative infrequency of IT, even the largest case series published to date comprise only a few hundred patients. Results from notable single-center patient series are summarized in **Tables 1** and **2**. More recently published series are sparse but have demonstrated excellent results; in a cohort of 25 patients receiving isolated ITs from 2010 to 2016, Beduschi and colleagues[28] have achieved 100% survival, calling for consideration of more preemptive transplantation, because this was superior to survival rates typically associated with long-term PN therapy.

The largest repository of outcomes data comes from the ITR, an organization that pools the collective experience and outcomes of all centers performing IT. In the most recent registry report published by the ITR, 2699 recipients from 82 programs were analyzed, which found the overall survival rates for patients transplanted since 2000 were 77%, 58%, and 41% at 1 year, 5 years, and 10 years, respectively. At 6-month follow up, two-thirds of patients had become independent of PN therapy.[16]

Infection

Postoperatively, infection remains the most common complication, reported in up to 97% of patients,[24] and remains the most common cause of graft loss overall.[16] Bacterial infections account for the majority, perhaps due to the presence of intraluminal microbes in the graft and bacterial translocation in the setting of profound immunosuppression and/or graft injury. In the series of 500 ITs by Abu-Elmagd and

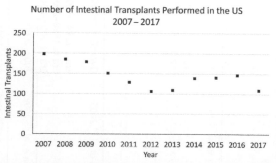

Fig. 3. Organ Procurement and Transplantation Network data demonstrating the number of ITs performed nationally from 2007–2017. (*Data from* Health Resources and Services Administration contract 234-2005-37011C.)

Table 1
Comparison of overall survival after intestinal transplant in notable single-center series

Study	Transplant Period	N	Overall Patient Survival	Significant Associations with Improved Patient Survival
Abu-Elmagd et al,[22] 2009	Overall: 1990–2003	453	85%, 61%, 42%, and 35% at 1 y, 5 y, 10 y, and 15 y, respectively	• Early transplant (<12 mo on PN) • Patient age 2–18 y • Combined intestinal-liver grafts • Addition of induction to immunosuppression • More recent transplant era
	Era I: 1990–1994	62	40% at 5 y	
	Era II: 1995–2001	106	56% at 5 y	
	Era III: 2000–2003	285	68% at 5 y	
Farmer et al,[23] 2010	Overall: 1991–2010	88	80%, 70%, and 65% at 1 y, 3 y, and 5 y, respectively	• Combined intestinal-liver grafts • PRA <20% • Absence of DSAs • Warm ischemia time <1 h • Cold ischemia time <10 h • Negative T-cell crossmatch • Use of IL2RA induction • Recipient spleen conservation • More recent transplant era
	Era I: 1991–2000	N/A	N/A	
	Era II: 2001–2010	N/A	N/A	
Tzakis et al,[24] 2005	Overall: 1994–2005	98	65%, 49%, and 49% at 1 y, 3 y, and 5 y, respectively	• Patient living outside hospital before transplant • More recent transplant era
	Era I: 1994–1997	N/A	44% and 25%	
	Era II: 1998–2000	N/A	56% and 44%	
	Era III: 2001–2005	N/A	73% and 58% at 1 y and 3 y, respectively	
Vianna et al,[25] 2009	2003–2009	106	77.5%, 56.9%, and 57% at 1 y, 5 y, and 10 y, respectively	• Use of isolated intestinal graft (over multivisceral graft)
Langnas et al,[26] 2000	1990–2001	106	70% at 2 y	n/a
Goulet et al,[27] 2005	1994–2004	52	71.5% at 3 y	• Use of IL2RA induction • Fewer surgeries prior to transplant • Home PN (vs in hospital) prior to transplant

Abbreviations: IL2RA, interleukin-2 receptor antagonist; N, number of patients; N/A, data not available; PRA, panel-reactive antibody.

Table 2
Comparison of common long-term complications after intestinal transplant in notable single-center series

Study	Transplant Period	N	Infection Rate, Related Deaths	Required Retransplantation	Post-transplant Lymphoproliferative Disease, n (%)	Graft-Versus-Host Disease, n (%)	CytomegaloVirus Infection, n (%)
Abu- Elmagd et al,[22] 2009	1990–2003	453	N/A, 54	73/215 (intestine only) 7/142 (liver-intestine) 9/113 (multivisceral)	57 (13)	38 (8.3)	83 (18)
Tzakis et al,[24] 2005	1994–2005	98	97%, 17	7/98	7 (7.1)	6 (6.1)	N/A
Vianna et al,[25] 2009	2003–2009	106	N/A, 14	N/A	4 (3.7)	7 (6.6)	6 (5.7)
Langnas et al,[26] 2000	1990–2001	106	93%, N/A	N/A	10 (9.4)	N/A	16 (15)
Goulet et al,[27] 2005	1994–2004	52	N/A, 10	4/52	12 (23)	N/A	11 (21)

Abbreviations: Infection Rate, percent of patients experiencing any infection postoperatively; Infection-related Deaths, any death attributed to bacterial, viral, or fungal sepsis; n, number of patients; N/A, data not available; Retransplantation, number of patients who required removal of graft and received a second transplant.

colleagues,[22,23] 54 fatal infections were reported; 61% were bacterial, 31% were fungal, and 7% were viral in etiology. Although often not fatal, approximately 40% of IT recipients develop a viral enteritis in their postoperative course.[29] The most frequently implicated viruses include cytomegalovirus, adenovirus, calicivirus, and rotavirus.[29–32] When considering enteritis as a diagnosis, however, it is essential to also rule out allograft rejection with endoscopy and biopsy, because both may have similar clinical presentations but require opposite alterations in immunosuppression for treatment.[33,34]

Rejection

Intestinal allografts are particularly sensitive to rejection in comparison to other organs. Early series have reported the incidence of acute cellular rejection in 50% to 75% of patients, with treatment refractory episodes in 9% of cases.[22] Repopulation of the intestine allograft by recipient T and B lymphocytes has been demonstrated over a period of several weeks after transplant.[35] Although this process is observed in other transplanted organs, it is postulated that the resulting alloimmune responses are greater in IT recipients due to the large amount of mucosal associated lymphoid tissue, high cell turnover, bacterial colonization, and vascularity unique to intestinal grafts.[36] The ITR reports graft survival after 1 year has not appreciably improved over the past decade, with overall rates of 71%, 50%, and 41% at 1 year, 5 years, and 10 years respectively. Although sepsis accounts for more than 50% of graft losses (often related to heavy immunosuppression to prevent or treat of allograft rejection), rejection is the primary cause of graft loss in 13%.[16]

Recent investigation has focused on antibody-mediated rejection (AMR) in IT and the role of donor-specific antibodies (DSAs). These HLA-binding antibodies can exist prior to transplant or develop de novo after transplantation and may persist after immunosuppression. Patients with persistent DSAs after IT have approximately double the risk of acute humoral rejection, and chronic rejection is significantly associated with either persistent DSAs or de novo DSAs after transplantation.[36] Combined transplantation with a liver graft is protective in this regard, because these patients are more likely to clear preformed DSAs. Cheng and colleagues[37] demonstrated a 25% prevalence of de novo DSAs in IT patients and found that patients with mismatch in the HLA-DQ locus were more likely to develop DSAs de novo.

Non-HLA antibodies have also been implicated in rejection of ITs. Gerlach and colleagues[38] showed that patients who developed antibodies against the angiotensin II type I receptor and the endothelin type A receptor had higher rates of graft rejection than those who did not (80% vs 55%). Like DSAs, these non-HLA antibodies may be preexisting, may develop de novo, and are more likely in patients with a greater number of HLA class II mismatches. Formation of non-HLA antibodies has been observed to precede development of HLA class II DSAs, suggesting that they may act as triggers to a more robust DSA-mediated allogenic response; however, further investigation is needed to clearly elucidate this mechanism and its role in AMR.

Chronic Kidney Disease

Chronic kidney disease (CKD) is a well-known complication after nonrenal solid organ transplants and, of all organs, CKD is most prevalent among IT recipients.[39] The association is primarily attributed to nephrotoxicity secondary to calcineurin inhibitor immunosuppression, which is required in greater doses for IT than other solid organ allografts. Huard and colleagues[40] reviewed a cohort of 843 adult patients from the Scientific Registry of Transplant Recipients and found CKD occurred in 25% at 5 years, and development of CKD carried a 6-fold increase in mortality. Incorporation of induction therapy, which is now standard practice, has been shown to be a protective factor, presumably due to the lower doses of calcineurin inhibitors required. In comparing immunosuppression regimens, tacrolimus-based therapy carries decreased CKD risk compared with cyclosporine-based protocols.

Post-transplant Lymphoproliferative Disease

Post-transplant lymphoproliferative disease (PTLD) is a malignant complication of transplantation characterized by uncontrolled B-cell proliferation, most often due to activation of latent Epstein-Barr virus infection in the context of immunosuppression. Rates of PTLD are highest in IT patients, occurring in 5% to 23% of IT recipients.[22,24–27,41] Higher rates of PTLD for IT recipients are likely due to both the increased immunosuppression and the greater mass of transplanted lymphoid tissue associated with intestinal grafts.[42] The initial treatment of PTLD typically consists of a reduction in immunosuppression to bolster T-cell responses. If this fails, rituximab is second-line therapy and yields response rates in greater than 50% of patients.[43,44] Ultimately for patients who do not respond to these measures, addition of CHOP-based chemotherapy is warranted although carries an increased treatment-related mortality in the realm of 10%.[42]

Graft-Versus-Host Disease

IT carries the potential drawback GVHD in 5% to 10% patients[20,45] due to the large quantity of mature donor lymphocytes present in the graft. These donor lymphocytes can trigger immune responses in the recipient with devastating consequences. There are variable mortality rates from GVHD reported by individual centers. In the series by Mazariegos and colleagues,[45] 2 of 14 patients with GVHD died, whereas Wu and colleagues[20] noted that patients with GVHD had 77% mortality during their follow-up period. Clinical features include macular skin rash with blistering, oral lesions, diarrhea, and cytopenia secondary to marrow suppression. GVHD is more likely to occur in pediatric patients, recipients who have undergone splenectomy, and those receiving multivisceral transplants, in particular grafts, including spleen.[20]

FUTURE DIRECTIONS
Novel Preservation Techniques

As with most organs, standard preservation techniques for ITs have not evolved appreciably beyond vascular cannulation with cold perfusate and static cold storage. Of the abdominal organs, intestinal grafts are the most susceptible to preservation injury and have a recommended maximum cold ischemia time of 6 hours to 8 hours.[46] The mucosa is the most vulnerable component of the graft and histologically demonstrates multifocal basement membrane separation and submucosal edema within the first 6 hours of preservation.[47,48] Intraluminal instillation of preservation solutions has been shown to improve tissue morphology and reduce mucosal edema in human and animal models, although large randomized trials to compare their effect on patient outcomes are lacking.[49,50] In a small series of 5 transplants, Munoz-Abraham and colleagues[51] have shown efficacy of a hypothermic extracorporeal perfusion system that circulated continuous perfusate through both the vasculature and luminal surfaces of the graft, resulting in favorable histopathologic changes compared with static cold preservation. At many US centers, preservation with University of Wisconsin solution remains the gold standard, although numerous alternatives have been used and are reviewed elsewhere.[47,49]

With the advent of normothermic machine perfusion (NMP) systems in other organs, which have now demonstrated clinical feasibility, comparable immediate outcomes, and lower rates of graft injury,[52–54] the use of NMP in IT remains to be explored. Given that intestinal grafts are more sensitive to cold storage and ischemia, it could be postulated that NMP technology, which uses oxygenated blood as a perfusate, might be of particular benefit in this population. To the authors' knowledge, there have been no reports to date of clinical NMP use for IT.

Strategies for Managing Donor-specific Antibody

Because DSAs are prevalent among IT recipients, strategies continue to evolve to counteract AMR. Traditionally, desensitization protocols used combinations of intravenous immunoglobulin (IVIG) and plasmapheresis to reduce pretransplant panel-reactive antibody levels.[51,55] Although this approach enables earlier transplant without acute rejection, the effects are short lived due to persistence of antibody-producing B cells and plasma cells in these patients.[56,57] In the series by Abu-Elmagd and colleagues,[36] 39% of IT patients with preformed DSAs who received IVIG had persistent antibodies. New advances in desensitization have incorporated rituximab[58] as well as the protease inhibitor bortezomib,[59] in an aim to suppress B cells and plasma cells, respectively; however, HLA antibodies may continue to persist or rebound after initial response due to compensatory B-cell and T-helper cell expansion in germinal centers.[60] Kwun and colleagues[61] have recently demonstrated that the addition of costimulation blockade with belatacept (anti-CD152) to a regimen with bortezomib (so-called dual targeting) results in more sustained desensitization and rejection-free survival in nonhuman primates undergoing renal transplants.

Alternative strategies to reduce AMR have also focused on modulation of the complement pathway. The monoclonal antibody against C5, eculizumab, has been successfully used following IT to prevent AMR in a sensitized patient who had previously rejected 2 grafts.[62] Vo and colleagues[63] verified the safety and efficacy of C1 esterase inhibitor (C1-INH) in a placebo-controlled trial of renal transplant patients and saw decreased levels of C1q-positive DSAs among C1-INH recipients. They also noted fewer episodes of delayed graft function in these patients, possibly related to the favorable impact of complement inhibition on ischemia-reperfusion injury.[63,64] Although neither C1-INH or eculizumab has met US Food and Drug Administration approval to treat or prevent allograft rejection, both have potential to change the standard of care in managing patients with preformed or de novo alloantibodies.

SUMMARY

IT is a complex procedure for the treatment of IF in patients who fail PN therapy. Isolated small bowel grafts are the most commonly transplanted, but intestine grafts may be combined with other intra-abdominal organs on a shared vascular pedicle. In comparison with other transplanted organs, ITs are highly immunogenic due to the large burden of transplanted lymphoid tissue, high cellular turnover, and presence of intraluminal microbiota. These features place patients at increased risk to develop immunosuppression-related complications, namely cellular rejection and AMR, infection, kidney disease, lymphoproliferative disorders, and GVHD. New advances in immunosuppression, in particular those aimed at desensitization of the humoral response, will continue to make IT a more acceptable, life-saving procedure in appropriately selected patients.

REFERENCES

1. Kappus M, Diamond S, Hurt RT, et al. Intestinal failure: new definition and clinical implications. Curr Gastroenterol Rep 2016;18(9):48.

2. O'Keefe SJ, Buchman AL, Fishbein TM, et al. Short bowel syndrome and intestinal failure: consensus definitions and overview. Clin Gastroenterol Hepatol 2006; 4(1):6–10.

3. Pironi L, Konrad D, Brandt C, et al. Clinical classification of adult patients with chronic intestinal failure due to benign disease: an international multicenter cross-sectional survey. Clin Nutr 2018;37(2):728–38.

4. Crenn P, Messing B, Cynober L. Citrulline as a biomarker of intestinal failure due to enterocyte mass reduction. Clin Nutr 2008;27(3):328–39.

5. Fjermestad H, Hvistendahl M, Jeppesen PB. Fasting and postprandial plasma citrulline and the correlation to intestinal function evaluated by 72-hour metabolic balance studies in short bowel jejunostomy patients with intestinal failure. JPEN J Parenter Enteral Nutr 2017. 148607116687497.

6. Jeppesen PB, Mortensen PB. Intestinal failure defined by measurements of intestinal energy and wet weight absorption. Gut 2000;46(5):701–6.

7. Fonseca G, Burgermaster M, Larson E, et al. The relationship between parenteral nutrition and central line-associated bloodstream infections: 2009-2014. JPEN J Parenter Enteral Nutr 2018;42(1):171–5.

8. Barco S, Heuschen CB, Salman B, et al. Home parenteral nutrition-associated thromboembolic and bleeding events: results of a cohort study of 236 individuals. J Thromb Haemost 2016;14(7):1364–73.

9. Gonzalez-Hernandez J, Daoud Y, Styers J, et al. Central venous thrombosis in children with intestinal failure on long-term parenteral nutrition. J Pediatr Surg 2016;51(5):790–3.

10. Kelly DA. Intestinal failure-associated liver disease: what do we know today? Gastroenterology 2006;130(2 Suppl 1):S70–7.

11. Pironi L, Goulet O, Buchman A, et al. Outcome on home parenteral nutrition for benign intestinal failure: a review of the literature and benchmarking with the European prospective survey of ESPEN. Clin Nutr 2012;31(6):831–45.

12. National Coverage Determination (NCD) for intestinal and multi-visceral transplantation (260.5). 2006. Accessed June 2, 2018.

13. Vianna RM, Mangus RS, Kubal C, et al. Multivisceral transplantation for diffuse portomesenteric thrombosis. Ann Surg 2012;255(6):1144–50.

14. Mangus RS, Tector AJ, Kubal CA, et al. Multivisceral transplantation: expanding indications and improving outcomes. J Gastrointest Surg 2013;17(1):179–86 [discussion: p 186–7].

15. Rege AS, Sudan DL. Autologous gastrointestinal reconstruction: review of the optimal nontransplant surgical options for adults and children with short bowel syndrome. Nutr Clin Pract 2013;28(1):65–74.

16. Grant D, Abu-Elmagd K, Mazariegos G, et al. Intestinal transplant registry report: global activity and trends. Am J Transplant 2015;15(1):210–9.

17. Matsumoto CS, Kaufman SS, Fishbein TM. Inclusion of the colon in intestinal transplantation. Curr Opin Organ Transplant 2011;16(3):312–5.

18. Sudan DL, Iyer KR, Deroover A, et al. A new technique for combined liver/small intestinal transplantation. Transplantation 2001;72(11):1846–8.

19. Kato T, Tzakis AG, Selvaggi G, et al. Transplantation of the spleen: effect of splenic allograft in human multivisceral transplantation. Ann Surg 2007;246(3): 436–44 [discussion: 445–436].

20. Wu G, Selvaggi G, Nishida S, et al. Graft-versus-host disease after intestinal and multivisceral transplantation. Transplantation 2011;91(2):219–24.

21. Hawksworth JS, Desai CS, Khan KM, et al. Visceral transplantation in patients with intestinal-failure associated liver disease: evolving indications, graft selection, and outcomes. Am J Transplant 2018;18(6):1312–20.

22. Abu-Elmagd KM, Costa G, Bond GJ, et al. Five hundred intestinal and multivisceral transplantations at a single center: major advances with new challenges. Ann Surg 2009;250(4):567–81.

23. Farmer DG, Venick RS, Colangelo J, et al. Pretransplant predictors of survival after intestinal transplantation: analysis of a single-center experience of more than 100 transplants. Transplantation 2010;90(12):1574–80.

24. Tzakis AG, Kato T, Levi DM, et al. 100 multivisceral transplants at a single center. Ann Surg 2005;242(4):480–90 [discussion: 491–3].

25. Vianna R, Kubal C, Mangus R, et al. Intestinal and multivisceral transplantation at Indiana University: 6 years' experience with 100 cases. Clin Transplant 2009;219–28.

26. Langnas AN, Sudan DL, Kaufman S, et al. Intestinal transplantation: a single-center experience. Transplant Proc 2000;32(6):1228.

27. Goulet O, Sauvat F, Ruemmele F, et al. Results of the Paris program: ten years of pediatric intestinal transplantation. Transplant Proc 2005;37(4):1667–70.

28. Beduschi T, Garcia J, Farag A, et al. Breaking the 5 year mark with 100% survival for intestinal transplant -time to become protagonist in the management of intestinal failure? Transplantation 2017;101(6S2):S136.

29. Ziring D, Tran R, Edelstein S, et al. Infectious enteritis after intestinal transplantation: incidence, timing, and outcome. Transplant Proc 2004;36(2):379–80.

30. Pinchoff RJ, Kaufman SS, Magid MS, et al. Adenovirus infection in pediatric small bowel transplantation recipients. Transplantation 2003;76(1):183–9.

31. Adeyi OA, Costa G, Abu-Elmagd KM, et al. Rotavirus infection in adult small intestine allografts: a clinicopathological study of a cohort of 23 patients. Am J Transplant 2010;10(12):2683–9.

32. Kaufman SS, Chatterjee NK, Fuschino ME, et al. Calicivirus enteritis in an intestinal transplant recipient. Am J Transpl 2003;3(6):764–8.

33. Rege A, Sudan D. Intestinal transplantation. Best Pract Res Clin Gastroenterol 2016;30(2):319–35.

34. Fishbein TM. Intestinal transplantation. N Engl J Med 2009;361(10):998–1008.

35. Iwaki Y, Starzl TE, Yagihashi A, et al. Replacement of donor lymphoid tissue in small-bowel transplants. Lancet 1991;337(8745):818–9.

36. Abu-Elmagd KM, Wu G, Costa G, et al. Preformed and de novo donor specific antibodies in visceral transplantation: long-term outcome with special reference to the liver. Am J Transplant 2012;12(11):3047–60.

37. Cheng EY, Everly MJ, Kaneku H, et al. Prevalence and clinical impact of donor-specific alloantibody among intestinal transplant recipients. Transplantation 2017;101(4):873–82.

38. Gerlach UA, Lachmann N, Ranucci G, et al. Non-HLA antibodies may accelerate immune responses after intestinal and multivisceral transplantation. Transplantation 2017;101(1):141–9.

39. Ojo AO, Held PJ, Port FK, et al. Chronic renal failure after transplantation of a nonrenal organ. N Engl J Med 2003;349(10):931–40.

40. Huard G, Iyer K, Moon J, et al. The high incidence of severe chronic kidney disease after intestinal transplantation and its impact on patient and graft survival. Clin Transplant 2017;31(5).

41. Reyes J, Green M, Bueno J, et al. Epstein Barr virus associated posttransplant lymphoproliferative disease after intestinal transplantation. Transplant Proc 1996;28(5):2768–9.
42. Dharnidharka VR, Webster AC, Martinez OM, et al. Post-transplant lymphoproliferative disorders. Nat Rev Dis Primers 2016;2:15088.
43. Oertel SH, Verschuuren E, Reinke P, et al. Effect of anti-CD 20 antibody rituximab in patients with post-transplant lymphoproliferative disorder (PTLD). Am J Transplant 2005;5(12):2901–6.
44. Berney T, Delis S, Kato T, et al. Successful treatment of posttransplant lymphoproliferative disease with prolonged rituximab treatment in intestinal transplant recipients. Transplantation 2002;74(7):1000–6.
45. Mazariegos GV, Abu-Elmagd K, Jaffe R, et al. Graft versus host disease in intestinal transplantation. Am J Transplant 2004;4(9):1459–65.
46. Wei L, Hata K, Doorschodt BM, et al. Experimental small bowel preservation using Polysol: a new alternative to University of Wisconsin solution, Celsior and histidine-tryptophan-ketoglutarate solution? World J Gastroenterol 2007;13(27): 3684–91.
47. Oltean M, Churchill TA. Organ-specific solutions and strategies for the intestinal preservation. Int Rev Immunol 2014;33(3):234–44.
48. Tesi RJ, Jaffe BM, McBride V, et al. Histopathologic changes in human small intestine during storage in Viaspan organ preservation solution. Arch Pathol Lab Med 1997;121(7):714–8.
49. Roskott AM, Nieuwenhuijs VB, Dijkstra G, et al. Small bowel preservation for intestinal transplantation: a review. Transpl Int 2011;24(2):107–31.
50. Trentadue G, van Praagh J, Olinga P, et al. Luminal preservation of the human small bowel graft reduces mucosal damage during cold storage. Transplantation 2017;101(6S2):S80.
51. Gondolesi G, Blondeau B, Maurette R, et al. Pretransplant immunomodulation of highly sensitized small bowel transplant candidates with intravenous immune globulin. Transplantation 2006;81(12):1743–6.
52. Iyer A, Gao L, Doyle A, et al. Normothermic ex vivo perfusion provides superior organ preservation and enables viability assessment of hearts from DCD donors. Am J Transplant 2015;15(2):371–80.
53. Warnecke G, Van Raemdonck D, Smith MA, et al. Normothermic ex-vivo preservation with the portable Organ Care System Lung device for bilateral lung transplantation (INSPIRE): a randomised, open-label, non-inferiority, phase 3 study. Lancet Respir Med 2018;6(5):357–67.
54. Nasralla D, Coussios CC, Mergental H, et al. A randomized trial of normothermic preservation in liver transplantation. Nature 2018;557(7703):50–+.
55. Jordan SC, Vo AA, Peng A, et al. Intravenous gammaglobulin (IVIG): A novel approach to improve transplant rates and outcomes in highly HLA-sensitized patients. Am J Transplant 2006;6(3):459–66.
56. Jordan SC, Reinsmoen N, Lai CH, et al. Novel immunotherapeutic approaches to improve rates and outcomes of transplantation in sensitized renal allograft recipients. Discov Med 2012;13(70):235–45.
57. Berger M, Zeevi A, Farmer DG, et al. Immunologic challenges in small bowel transplantation. Am J Transplant 2012;12:S2–8.
58. Vo AA, Lukovsky M, Toyoda M, et al. Rituximab and intravenous immune globulin for desensitization during renal transplantation. N Engl J Med 2008;359(3): 242–51.

59. Gerlach UA, Schoenemann C, Lachmann N, et al. Salvage therapy for refractory rejection and persistence of donor-specific antibodies after intestinal transplantation using the proteasome inhibitor bortezomib. Transpl Int 2011;24(5):e43–5.

60. Kwun J, Burghuber C, Manook M, et al. Humoral compensation after bortezomib treatment of allosensitized recipients. J Am Soc Nephrol 2017;28(7):1991–6.

61. Kwun J, Burghuber C, Manook M, et al. Successful desensitization with proteasome inhibition and costimulation blockade in sensitized nonhuman primates. Blood Adv 2017;1(24):2115–9.

62. Fan J, Tryphonopoulos P, Tekin A, et al. Eculizumab salvage therapy for antibody-mediated rejection in a desensitization-resistant intestinal re-transplant patient. Am J Transplant 2015;15(7):1995–2000.

63. Vo AA, Zeevi A, Choi J, et al. A phase I/II placebo-controlled trial of C1-inhibitor for prevention of antibody-mediated rejection in HLA sensitized patients. Transplantation 2015;99(2):299–308.

64. Castellano G, Melchiorre R, Loverre A, et al. Therapeutic targeting of classical and lectin pathways of complement protects from ischemia-reperfusion-induced renal damage. Am J Pathol 2010;176(4):1648–59.

Is This Organ Donor Safe?

Donor-Derived Infections in Solid Organ Transplantation

Staci A. Fischer, MD[a,b,*]

KEYWORDS

- Transplant infections • Donor-transmitted infections • Donor-derived infections
- Organ donor screening • Lymphocytic choriomeningitis virus

KEY POINTS

- Organ donor–derived infections are uncommon but may cause significant morbidity and mortality in transplant recipients.
- Diagnosis of infection in deceased donors may be challenging due to reliance on next of kin to provide critical medical and social history, the short time available for evaluation and testing, and the lack of rapid, sensitive assays for uncommon organisms.
- Growing experience with the use of donors at increased risk for infection with human immunodeficiency virus, hepatitis B virus, and hepatitis C virus suggests that these donors may be used with caution and informed consent of the recipients.
- Donors with unrecognized meningoencephalitis may transmit multiple infections including viruses, for which limited therapies exist.
- Careful screening of donors is paramount to improving the safety of organ transplantation.

In 2017, more than 10,000 deceased donors provided organs for more than 28,000 patients in the United States.[1] Although advances in critical care and immunosuppressive therapy have facilitated the use of more deceased donors and improved the outcomes of many transplant procedures, infection remains a common and significant complication of solid organ transplantation (SOT).[2] Causes of post-transplant infection include health care–associated infection during hospitalizations, community-acquired infection, and reactivation of latent infection in the recipient. Transmission of infection from donor to recipient, although less common than the other etiologies, ranges from the routine to the devastating. Although donor-derived infections, such as

This article originally appeared in Infectious Diseases Clinics of North America, Volume 32, Issue 3, September 2018.
Disclosure Statement: The author has nothing to disclose.
[a] The Warren Alpert Medical School of Brown University, 222 Richmond Street, Providence, RI 02903, USA; [b] Accreditation Council for Graduate Medical Education, 401 North Michigan Avenue, Suite 2000, Chicago, IL 60611, USA
* 470 North Lane, Bristol, RI 02809.
E-mail address: sfischer@acgme.org

Surg Clin N Am 99 (2019) 117–128
https://doi.org/10.1016/j.suc.2018.09.009
0039-6109/19/© 2018 Elsevier Inc. All rights reserved.

cytomegalovirus (CMV), are well-studied, anticipated, and able to be prevented in most cases, the number and variety of pathogens transmitted with transplantation continue to grow (**Box 1**).[3–31]

RISK OF INFECTION IN ORGAN DONORS

Most organs transplanted in the United States are from deceased donors, who often require intensive medical care prior to becoming candidates for donation, with mechanical ventilation, indwelling vascular and urinary catheters, and administration of broad-spectrum antimicrobials. As a result of intensive care, donors may become colonized or infected with resistant bacterial pathogens as well as fungi, including *Candida* and *Aspergillus*. In many cases, donors with documented bacterial infections on effective antimicrobial therapy may be used when the recipients are also treated; caution should be used with multidrug resistant organisms and infections of the allograft itself. Donors may also harbor latent infections (eg, *Histoplasma*, *Coccidioides immitis*, *Mycobacterium tuberculosis*, and strongyloidiasis), based on their epidemiologic exposures. When transplanted into a recipient on immunosuppressive therapy, these latent infections may reactivate, causing disseminated disease. Because 1 donor may provide organs to as many as 8 recipients, who may be scattered across multiple transplant centers, states, and regions, prompt recognition of donor-derived infections and communication between transplant centers and organ procurement organizations (OPOs) is critical to improving outcomes of these often devastating infections.

WHEN TO SUSPECT DONOR-DERIVED INFECTION

In most cases, infections transmitted from an organ donor present early post-transplant, often in the first 6 weeks. Some pathogens with long incubation periods or latent infection, however, may take months to even years to present in the immuno-compromised transplant recipient. Most outbreaks of infection have been identified when more than one recipient of an organ from a common deceased donor develops similar symptoms and signs.[8–12] Because recipients are often hospitalized in different transplant centers and may be under the care of different teams within the same institution, recognition of a pattern of clinical findings may be difficult. If a recipient develops fever, leukocytosis, leukopenia, or other potential signs of infection early post-transplant, and donor-derived infection is considered a possibility, the responsible OPO should be contacted to discuss the findings and determine whether other recipients of organs from the same donor are experiencing similar illnesses. State public health departments and the Centers for Disease Control and Prevention (CDC) can also be of assistance in investigating the cause of an outbreak of infection.

SCREENING ORGAN DONORS FOR INFECTION

Screening potential donors for infection remains crucial to improving the safety of organ transplantation. The United Network for Organ Sharing is contracted by the Department of Health and Human Services to serve as the Organ Procurement and Transplantation Network (OPTN), responsible for policy development and oversight of SOT in the United States. The policies of the OPTN and the experience of the transplant infectious disease community have resulted in recommendations for routine screening of potential donors for several pathogens (**Box 2**).[32–35] Screening for antibodies to HTLV types I and II had been routine for many years, but with the prevalence

Box 1
Pathogens reported to be transmitted via solid organ transplantation

<u>Bacteria</u>

Acinetobacter species

Bartonella species

Brucella species

Ehrlichia species

Enterobacter species

Enterococcus species

Escherichia coli

Klebsiella species

Legionella pneumophila

Listeria monocytogenes

Mycoplasma hominis

Nocardia species

Pseudomonas aeruginosa

Salmonella species

Serratia species

Staphylococcus aureus

Streptococcus species

Treponema pallidum

Veillonella species

Yersinia enterocolitica

<u>Fungi</u>

Aspergillus species

Blastomyces dermatiditis

Candida species

Coccidioides immitis

Cryptococcus neoformans

Histoplasma capsulatum

Prototheca

Scedosporium apiospermum

Zygomyces

Microsporidia

Encephalitozoon cuniculi

<u>Mycobacteria</u>

Mycobacterium tuberculosis

Nontuberculous *Mycobacteria*

<u>Parasites/protozoa/prions/amebae</u>

Babesia species

Balamuthia mandrillaris

Creutzfeld-Jakob disease

Naegleria fowleri

Plasmodium species

Schistosoma species

Strongyloides stercoralis

Toxoplasma gondii

Trypanosoma cruzi

Viruses

Adenovirus

BK virus

CMV

Epstein-Barr virus

HBV

HCV

Hepatitis D virus

Hepatitis E virus

Human herpesvirus 6

Human herpesvirus 7

Human herpesvirus 8

HIV

Human T-lymphotropic virus

Influenza virus

Lymphocytic choriomeningitis virus

Parainfluenza virus

Parvovirus B19

Rabies virus

Varicella-zoster virus

West Nile virus

Data from Refs.[3–31]

of infection in the United States and few donor-transmitted events, serologic screening for this viral pathogen is no longer indicated.[36]

All potential donors should be screened for blood-borne pathogens, such as HIV, hepatitis B, and hepatitis C; those living in endemic areas should also be tested for hepatitis E, an increasingly recognized pathogen in transplant recipients. Serology for CMV and Epstein-Barr virus should be performed to predict the risk of transmission and guide post-transplantation monitoring and CMV prophylaxis. Donors with specific epidemiologic risk factors for infection with endemic fungi, *Strongyloides*, *Trypanosoma cruzi*, *Cryptococcus*, West Nile virus, and other pathogens should be screened for infection with these organisms; in some cases, prophylactic therapy may be

---

Box 2
General screening for potential organ donors

Required by OPTN policy
  Serology for HIV, hepatitis B, and hepatitis C (repeat within 28 days of donation in living
  donors)
  CMV IgG
  Epstein-Barr virus IgG
  HIV-1/2 antibody or HIV antigen/antibody assay
  Hepatitis B surface antigen and core antibody; consider NAT
  Hepatitis C NAT
  Syphilis screening
  Toxoplasma IgG
  Blood, urine, and sputum cultures

Recommended additional screening:
  Tuberculosis screening (purified protein derivative or interferon-γ release assay)
  Testing based on prior history of living in an endemic area
    Strongyloides antibody
    Trypanosoma cruzi antibody
    Histoplasma antibody
    Blastomyces antibody
    Coccidioides immitis antibody
    Hepatitis E antibody
  Testing based on epidemiologic exposures
    Brucella antibody
    Cryptococcus antigen
    West Nile virus antibody

Organ-specific testing: urine culture for kidney donors, bronchoalveolar lavage fluid/sputum
culture for lung donors

Data from Refs.[32–35]

---

indicated.[18,31–35] The risk of infection is related to the tissue tropism of specific pathogens (eg, *Toxoplasma* and *Trypanosoma* in heart transplants and BK virus in kidney transplants) as well as viability of the organisms.

Because screening for many infections is based on serology, the sensitivity and specificity of the assays used must be considered in choosing a donor screening methodology. Results of these tests may also be affected by dilution from transfusion of multiple blood products and crystalloid into deceased donor candidates.

The key to assessing the risk of infection from a particular donor is obtaining an accurate history of exposures. OPOs are responsible for reviewing available medical records and interviewing family members to ascertain this information. Questionnaires used to guide next of kin discussions are not standardized across the United States but generally address medical and social factors to help assess organ quality and the risk of infection. The information gathered is dependent on the accurate knowledge of those questioned with the prospective donor's circumstances. In evaluating potential living donors, transplant centers have time to assess medical, social, and exposure histories and treat any identified infections prior to donation to prevent transmission.

SELECTED PATHOGENS THAT CAN BE DONOR TRANSMITTED
Balamuthia mandrillaris

Two outbreaks of donor-transmitted *Balamuthia mandrillaris* have recently been described.[20,21] This free-living ameba, known to cause granulomatous amebic encephalitis, is found in soil in multiple areas of the world, including the United States, where infection seems more common in patients of Hispanic ethnicity. Infection is believed to result from inhalation or inoculation into broken skin, with spread to the brain and spinal cord. In both transplant-related clusters, the organ donor presented with headache and focal brain lesions on CT or MRI; 1 donor had a several month history of neurologic symptoms. One donor had fever; the other was afebrile but demonstrated lymphocytic pleocytosis on cerebrospinal fluid (CSF) testing. In both cases, some recipients developed neurologic symptoms (eg, headache, blurred vision, and ataxia), whereas others were asymptomatic; fever was variably present. CSF revealed lymphocytic pleocytosis and MRI demonstrated multiple ring-enhancing lesions in some of the recipients. Histopathologic testing of brain tissue from symptomatic recipients at the CDC revealed evidence of *Balamuthia* infection, for which therapy was initiated with combinations of flucytosine, pentamidine, sulfadiazine, fluconazole, azithromycin, and miltefosine, with variable outcomes, including infection clearance, significant neurologic sequelae, and death.[21]

Coccidioides immitis

Coccidioides immitis is an endemic fungus in the southwestern United States, Mexico, and parts of Central and South America, which can be transmitted with transplantation. Deceased or living donors who have visited or lived in an endemic area may have viable organisms that reactivate in the setting of immunosuppression in the recipient, regardless of whether they or their families recall previous infection, which is usually asymptomatic. Guidelines for treatment of exposed recipients recommend fluconazole, 400 mg daily for 3 months to 12 months, for nonlung recipients and lifelong therapy for lung transplant recipients when the donor has evidence of pulmonary coccidioidomycosis.[34] Screening of potential donors from endemic areas has been recommended to guide informed consent and treatment of the recipients.

Lymphocytic Choriomeningitis Virus

Multiple outbreaks of donor-derived infection with lymphocytic choriomeningitis virus (LCMV) and related arenaviruses have been described in recent years.[8-10] Because infection is most commonly asymptomatic, recognition of donor infection is difficult. Some donors may present with aseptic meningitis; the timeframe for deciding whether to use a deceased donor generally precludes CSF testing (eg, by culture, polymerase chain reaction [PCR], and/or enzyme immunoassay), which is available through the CDC and some state health departments. Exposure to wild or pet mice or hamsters, which may harbor lifelong asymptomatic infection, may be an important clue to the possibility of LCMV infection, for which no screening tests are routinely available. Decreasing immunosuppressive therapy and administration of ribavirin may be of use in treating infected recipients, in whom the mortality rate has been high.[8,10]

Strongyloides stercoralis

Strongyloides stercoralis is endemic in tropical and subtropical areas, including the southern United States. Infection may be asymptomatic, with reactivation causing disseminated disease (termed, *hyperinfection syndrome*) in immunocompromised hosts. Most donor-derived infection cases present within the first 6 months after transplantation, with variable symptoms; fever and eosinophilia, hallmarks of infection in immunocompetent hosts, are often absent.[18,19] Screening donors who have traveled to or lived in endemic areas with serology may be useful in preventing infection, by treating the living donor prior to procurement and/or treating the recipients with ivermectin and/or albendazole.[19]

Trypanosoma cruzi

Chagas disease, caused by *Trypanosoma cruzi*, is endemic throughout much of Mexico, Central America, and South America. Several outbreaks of donor-derived infection have occurred in the United States.[17] The risk of transmission is highest in heart and intestine recipients, due to chronic infection of myocardial and enteric tissues, although recipients of liver and kidney transplants have also developed infection. Donors from endemic areas should be screened for infection with serologic testing, and caution used when considering heart or intestinal transplantation. Monitoring noncardiac recipients with PCR and serology may be of assistance in diagnosing donor-derived infection. Treatment with nifurtimox and/or benznidazole may be challenging in the United States, where these agents are not readily available.

USE OF DONORS AT RISK OF HEPATITIS B VIRUS, HEPATITIS C VIRUS, OR HUMAN IMMUNODEFICIENCY VIRUS INFECTION

Transplantation of organs from donors at risk for HIV, hepatitis B virus (HBV), and hepatitis C virus (HCV) poses inherent risk of transmission of infection to recipients. With increasingly effective therapies now available against these pathogens, centers are gaining experience with transplantation of organs from donors with treated (nonviremic) infection in selected recipients.[37–40]

All potential organ donors, regardless of risk, should undergo testing for HIV (anti-HIV 1/2 or HIV antigen/antibody), HBV (hepatitis B surface antigen and core antibody), and HCV (anti-HCV antibody and HCV-RNA by nucleic acid testing [NAT]), with results available prior to procurement. For potential living donors, testing should be repeated within 28 days of donation.

Although NAT has improved the sensitivity of testing potential organ donors for infection with these viruses, those with recent infection in the window period of current diagnostic testing may transmit infection. The US Public Health Service has developed guidelines for the testing and use of organs from donors at higher than average risk of infection with hepatitis B, hepatitis C, and HIV, which are termed, *increased risk donors (IRDs)* (**Box 3**).[41] It has been estimated that approximately 30% of donors in the United States and Canada meet these criteria.[42,43] As the opioid epidemic spreads in the US, more donors meet these criteria.

Those potential organ donors meeting criteria for increased risk should undergo more sensitive testing (eg, HIV NAT) prior to procurement, although results may not be available prior to transplantation from deceased donors. Living IRDs should undergo repeat testing using NAT within 28 days of surgery. Informed consent of recipients accepting organs from IRDs is critical, as is rigorous post-transplant NAT testing. Use of IRDs has been successful in many centers, proving an important resource in the current organ shortage. A recent registry review demonstrated a significant long-term survival benefit for recipients who accepted IRD kidneys, in which only 31% of those who declined an IRD offer had undergone transplant with a non-IRD donor after 5 years.[44]

MENINGOENCEPHALITIS

In recent years, outbreaks of donor-derived infections, such as rabies, West Nile virus, LCMV, and *Balamuthia*, have emphasized the difficulty in diagnosing encephalitis in potential deceased organ donors and the risk of transmission of infection if undetected (**Box 4**).[45,46] Donors with bacterial meningitis may be used if antimicrobial therapy is administered to the donor and all recipients. Undiagnosed meningoencephalitis of viral etiology may pose the greatest risk of donor-derived infection, due to high rates

Box 3
The US Public health service–defined increased risk donors

Men who have had sex with a man (MSM) in the past 12 months

Nonmedical injection drug use in the past 12 months

Having sex in exchange for money or drugs in the past 12 months

Having sex with a person known or suspected to have HIV, HBV, or HCV infection in the past 12 months

Women who have had sex with a man with a history of MSM behavior in the past 12 months

Having sex with a person who had sex in exchange for money or drugs in the past 12 months

Having sex with a person who injected drugs by intravenous, intramuscular, or subcutaneous routes for nonmedical purposes in the past 12 months

A child less than or equal to 18 months of age born to a mother known to be infected with or at increased risk for HIV, HBV, or HCV infection

A child who has been breastfed in the past 12 months whose mother is known to be infected with or at increased risk for HIV infection

In lockup, jail, prison, or a juvenile correctional facility for more than 72 consecutive hours in the past 12 months

Newly diagnosed with, or previously treated for, syphilis, gonorrhea, *Chlamydia*, or genital ulcers in the past 12 months

On hemodialysis in the past 12 months (HCV only)

When a deceased potential organ donor's medical/behavioral history cannot be obtained or risk factors cannot be determined, the donor should be considered at increased risk for HIV, HBV, and HCV infection because the donor's risk for infection is unknown.

When a deceased potential organ donor's blood specimen is hemodiluted, the donor should be considered at increased risk for HIV, HBV, and HCV infection because the donor's risk for infection is unknown.

From U.S. Department of Health & Human Services Organ Procurement and Transplantation Network. Understanding the risk of transmission of HIV, hepatitis B, and hepatitis C from PHS increased risk donors. Available at: https://optn.transplant.hrsa.gov/resources/guidance/understanding-hiv-hbv-hcv-risks-from-increased-risk-donors/. Accessed January 27, 2018.

Box 4
Central nervous system pathogens transmitted through solid organ transplantation

Aspergillus Species

Balamuthia mandrillaris

Coccidioides immitis

Cryptococcus neoformans

Herpes simplex virus

LCMV and related arenaviruses

Mycobacterium tuberculosis

Rabies virus

West Nile virus

of transmissibility, morbidity, and mortality and the lack of effective antiviral therapies. Recognition of infection may be limited by the myriad etiologies for fever and altered mental status in potential deceased organ donors as well as the limited diagnostic testing available for some of these pathogens (**Box 5**). Guidelines have been developed to assist OPOs in recognizing the potential donor with meningoencephalitis.[46]

When evaluating a potential donor with a presumed cerebrovascular accident (CVA) or stroke, OPOs and transplant centers should consider the following questions:

- Do the donor's age and comorbidities (eg, previous stroke, hypertension, and diabetes mellitus) support a diagnosis of CVA? Meningoencephalitis should be considered in younger donors and those without underlying comorbidities, in whom CVA is less likely.
- Were fever, altered mental status, and/or seizures noted on presentation? If there is not a clear explanation for these symptoms and signs, meningoencephalitis should be considered.
- Is there unexplained CSF pleocytosis, hypoglycorrhachia, or elevated protein (eg, no identified bacterial pathogen prior to initiation of antibacterial therapy)?
- Is there unexplained hydrocephalus, which could be a sign of infection?
- Is the donor immunosuppressed, so that the risk of infection is higher and atypical presentations possible?
- Does the donor have a history of potential environmental exposures to pathogens causing meningoencephalitis (eg, bats, rodents, and mosquitoes) or of living in areas endemic for or in the midst of epidemic spread of CNS pathogens (eg, West Nile virus and *Coccidioides*)?
- Was the donor homeless? This could result in exposure to rodents and their excreta.

In several investigations of transplant-related outbreaks of LCMV and rabies, risk factors for infection were not identified during pretransplant evaluation of the donors.[8,10,12] Caution should be used when the next of kin of a potential deceased donor is unfamiliar with the donor's recent history and exposures so that risk may not be accurately assessed.

INVESTIGATING AND REPORTING DONOR-DERIVED INFECTIONS

Prevention, identification, and treatment of potential donor-derived infections is a fundamental role of the transplant infectious disease specialist. The OPTN/UNOS, which regulates SOT in the United States, has an Ad Hoc Disease Transmission Advisory Committee (DTAC) that investigates possible transmission of infection and diseases (eg, malignancy) from donors to recipients and publishes its findings.[4–6,47]

Box 5
Challenges in recognizing central nervous system infections in potential deceased donors

Suspecting infection
  May be clinically silent
  May be difficult to differentiate from stroke or drug overdose

Diagnosing infection
  Limited time prior to procurement
  Specialized testing (eg, PCR) not available in a timely manner

Lack of effective treatments for many pathogens

When suspicious of donor-transmitted infection, notification of the responsible OPO and DTAC may help facilitate recognition of similar symptoms in other recipients and testing for possible donor-derived infections in the hope of improving outcomes of these uncommon events.

REFERENCES

1. U.S. Department of Health & Human Services Organ Procurement and Transplantation Network. Transplants by donor type. Available at: https://optn.transplant. hrsa.gov/data/view-data-reports/national-data/#. Accessed January 27, 2018.
2. Kotloff RM, Blosser S, Fulda GJ, et al. Management of the potential organ donor in the ICU: Society of Critical Care Medicine/American College of Chest Physicians/Association of Organ Procurement Organizations consensus statement. Crit Care Med 2015;43:1291–325.
3. Morris MI, Fischer SA, Ison MG. Infections transmitted by transplantation. Infect Dis Clin North Am 2010;24:497–514.
4. Ison MG, Grossi P, AST Infectious Diseases Community of Practice. Donor-derived infections in solid organ transplantation. Am J Transplant 2013;13:22–30.
5. Ison MG, Nalesnik MA. An update on donor-derived disease transmission in organ transplantation. Am J Transplant 2011;11:1123–30.
6. Ison MG, Hager J, Blumberg E, et al. Donor-derived disease transmission events in the United Stated: data reviewed by the OPTN/UNOS Disease Transmission Advisory Committee. Am J Transplant 2009;9:1929–35.
7. U.S. Department of Health & Human Services Organ Procurement and Transplantation Network. Pathogens of special interest. Available at: https://optn.transplant. hrsa.gov/media/1911/special_pathogens_list.pdf. Accessed January 27, 2018.
8. Fischer SA, Graham MB, Kuehnert MJ, et al. Transmission of lymphocytic choriomeningitis virus by organ transplantation. N Engl J Med 2006;354:2235–49.
9. Palacios G, Druce J, Du L, et al. A new arenavirus in a cluster of fatal transplant-associated diseases. N Engl J Med 2008;358:991–8.
10. Mathur G, Yadav K, Ford B, et al. High clinical suspicion of donor-derived disease leads to timely recognition and early intervention to treat solid organ transplant-transmitted lymphocytic choriomeningitis virus. Transpl Infect Dis 2017;19: e12707–15.
11. Iwamoto M, Jernigan DB, Guasch A, et al. Transmission of West Nile virus from an organ donor to four transplant recipients. N Engl J Med 2003;348:2196–203.
12. Srinivasan A, Burton EC, Kuehnert MJ, et al. Transmission of rabies virus from an organ donor to four transplant recipients. N Engl J Med 2005;352:1103–11.
13. Meije Y, Piersimoni C, Torre-Cisneros J, et al. Mycobacterial infections in solid organ transplant recipients. Clin Microbiol Infect 2014;20:89–101.
14. Kay A, Barry PM, Annambhotla P, et al. Solid organ transplant-transmitted tuberculosis linked to a community outbreak – California, 2015. Am J Transplant 2017; 17:2733–6.
15. Kusne S, Taranto S, Covington S, et al. Coccidioidomycosis transmission through organ transplantation: a report of the OPTN *Ad Hoc* disease transmission advisory committee. Am J Transplant 2016;16:3562–7.
16. Serody JS, Mill MR, Detterbeck FC, et al. Blastomycosis in transplant recipients: report of a case and review. Clin Infect Dis 1993;16:54–8.
17. Huprikar S, Bosserman E, Patel G, et al. Donor-derived *Trypanosoma cruzi* infection in solid organ recipients in the United States, 2001-2011. Am J Transplant 2013;13:2418–25.

18. Roxby AC, Gottlieb GS, Limaye AP. Strongyloidiasis in transplant patients. Clin Infect Dis 2009;49:1411–23.
19. Le M, Ravin K, Hasan A, et al. Single donor-derived strongyloidiasis in three solid organ transplant recipients: case series and review of the literature. Am J Transplant 2014;14:1199–206.
20. Centers for Disease Control and Prevention. *Balamuthia mandrillaris* transmitted through organ transplantation – Mississippi, 2009. Am J Transplant 2011;11: 173–6.
21. Farnon EC, Kokko KE, Budge PJ, et al. Transmission of *Balamuthia mandrillaris* by organ transplantation. Clin Infect Dis 2016;63:878–88.
22. Fischer SA. Emerging and rare viral infections in transplantation. In: Ljungman P, Snydman D, Boeckh M, editors. Transplant infections. 4th edition. Switzerland: Springer; 2016. p. 911–24.
23. Mirazo S, Ramos N, Mainardi V, et al. Transmission, diagnosis, and management of hepatitis E: an update. Hepat Med 2014;6:45–59.
24. Behrendt P, Steinmann E, Manns MP, et al. The impact of hepatitis E in the liver transplant setting. J Hepatol 2014;61:1418–29.
25. Kamar N, Garrouste C, Haagsma EB, et al. Factors associated with chronic hepatitis in patients with hepatitis E virus infection who have received solid organ transplants. Gastroenterology 2011;140:1481–9.
26. Schlosser B, Stein A, Neuhaus R, et al. Liver transplant from a donor with occult HEV infection induced chronic hepatitis and cirrhosis in the recipient. J Hepatol 2012;56:500–2.
27. Hocevar SN, Paddock CD, Spak CW, et al. Microsporidiosis acquired through solid organ transplantation: a public health investigation. Ann Intern Med 2014; 160:213–20.
28. Lion T. Adenovirus infections in immunocompetent and immunocompromised patients. Clin Microbiol Rev 2014;27:441–62.
29. Smibert OC, Wilson HL, Sohail A, et al. Donor-derived *Mycoplasma hominis* and an apparent cluster of *M. hominis* cases in solid organ transplant recipients. Clin Infect Dis 2017;65:1504–8.
30. Vora NM, Basavaraju SV, Feldman KA, et al. Racoon rabies virus variant transmission through solid organ transplantation. JAMA 2013;310:398–407.
31. Kauffman CA, Freifeld AG, Andes DR, et al. Endemic fungal infections in solid organ and hematopoietic cell transplant recipients enrolled in the Transplant-Associated Infection Surveillance Network (TRANSNET). Transpl Infect Dis 2014;16:213–24.
32. Len O, Garzoni C, Lumbreras C, et al. Recommendations for screening of donor and recipient prior to solid organ transplantation and to minimize transmission of donor-derived infections. Clin Microbiol Infect 2014;20:10–8.
33. Fischer SA, Lu K, American Society of Transplantation Infectious Diseases Community of Practice. Screening of donor and recipient in solid organ transplantation. Am J Transplant 2013;13:9–21.
34. Singh N, Huprikar S, Burdette SD, et al. Donor-derived fungal infections in organ transplant recipients: guidelines of the American Society of Transplantation, Infectious Diseases Community of Practice. Am J Transplant 2012;12:2414–28.
35. Levi ME, Kumar D, Green M, et al. Considerations for screening live kidney donors for endemic infections: a viewpoint on the UNOS policy. Am J Transplant 2014;14:1003–11.
36. US Department of Health & Human Services Organ Procurement and Transplantation Network. Guidance for HTLV-1/2 screening and confirmation in potential donors and

reporting potential HTLV-1 infection. Available at: https://optn.transplant.hrsa.gov/resources/guidance/guidance-for-htlv-1-screening-and-confirmation-in-potential-donors-and-reporting-potential-htlv-1-infection/. Accessed January 27, 2018.

37. Huprikar S, Danziger-Isakov L, Ahn J, et al. Solid organ transplantation from hepatitis B virus-positive donors: consensus guidelines for recipient management. Am J Transplant 2015;15:1162–72.

38. Levitsky J, Formica RN, Bloom RD, et al. The American Society of Transplantation consensus conference on the use of hepatitis C viremic donors in solid organ transplantation. Am J Transplant 2017;17:2790–802.

39. Muller E, Barday Z, Mendelson M, et al. HIV-positive-to-HIV-positive kidney transplantation – results at 3 to 5 years. N Engl J Med 2015;372:613–20.

40. Wright AJ, Rose C, Toews M, et al. An exception to the rule or a rule for the exception? The potential of using HIV-positive donors in Canada. Transplantation 2017; 101:671–4.

41. U.S. Department of Health & Human Services Organ Procurement and TransplantationNetwork. Understanding the risk of transmission of HIV, hepatitis B,and hepatitis C from PHS increased risk donors. Available at: https://optn.transplant.hrsa.gov/resources/guidance/understanding-hiv-hbv-hcv-risks-fromincreased-risk-donors/. Accessed January 27, 2018.

42. L'Huillier AG, Humar A, Payne C, et al. Organ utilization from increased infectious risk donors: an observational study. Transpl Infect Dis 2017;19:e12785–92.

43. Irwin L, Kotton CN, Elias N, et al. Utilization of increased risk for transmission of infectious disease donor organs in solid organ transplantation: retrospective analysis of disease transmission and safety. Transpl Infect Dis 2017;19:e12791–7.

44. Bowring MG, Holscher CM, Zhou S, et al. Turn down for what? Patient outcomes associated with declining increased infectious risk donors. Am J Transplant 2017;1–8. https://doi.org/10.1111/ajt.14577.

45. Basavaraju SV, Kuehnert MJ, Zaki SR, et al. Encephalitis caused by pathogens transmitted through organ transplants, United States, 2002-2013. Emerg Infect Dis 2014;20:1443–51.

46. U.S. Department of Health & Human Services Organ Procurement and Transplantation Network. Guidance for recognizing central nervous system infections in potential deceased organ donors. Available at: https://optn.transplant.hrsa.gov/resources/guidance/guidance-for-recognizing-central-nervous-system-infections-in-potential-deceased-organ-donors/. Accessed January 27, 2018.

47. U.S. Department of Health & Human Services Organ Procurement and Transplantation Network. Disease Transmission Advisory Committee. Available at: https://optn.transplant.hrsa.gov/members/committees/disease-transmission-advisory-committee/. Accessed January 27, 2018.

Composite and Multivisceral Transplantation

Nomenclature, Surgical Techniques, Current Practice, and Long-term Outcome

Guilherme Costa, MD[a], Neha Parekh, MS, RD[a],
Mohammed Osman, MD[a], Sherif Armanyous, MD[c],
Masato Fujiki, MD, PhD[a], Kareem Abu-Elmagd, MD, PhD[a,b,*]

KEYWORDS

- Liver-intestinal transplantation • Multivisceral transplantation
- Visceral transplantation • Intestinal failure • Portomesenteric venous thrombosis
- Surgical technique

KEY POINTS

- Composite and multivisceral transplantation is a life-saving procedure for patients with combined abdominal organ and gut failure.
- The observed continual improvement in survival outcome is the result of innovative surgical techniques, novel immunosuppressive protocols, and state-of-art postoperative care.
- Reestablishment of long-term nutritional autonomy with restored quality of life and socioeconomic milestones is achievable in most survivors.
- Further progress is anticipated with better in-depth understanding of innate immunity, adaptive gut alloimmunity, allograft tolerance, and the biology of gut microbiota.

INTRODUCTION

For nearly 4 decades, the abdominal viscera was considered a forbidden organ for clinical transplantation because of the associated massive lymphoid tissue, high antigenicity, and microbial colonization.[1,2] The late 1980s witnessed successful sporadic attempts under cyclosporine-based immunosuppression.[3] However, the

This article originally appeared in Gastroenterology Clinics of North America, Volume 47, Issue 2, June 2018.
Disclosure Statement: The authors have nothing to disclose.
[a] Center for Gut Rehabilitation and Transplantation, Cleveland Clinic, 9500 Euclid Avenue, Desk A100, Cleveland, OH 44195, USA; [b] Cleveland Clinic Lerner College of Medicine, Cleveland Clinic, 9500 Euclid Avenue, Desk A100, Cleveland, OH 44195, USA; [c] Department of Nephrology, Cleveland Clinic, 9500 Euclid Avenue, Desk A100, Cleveland, OH 44195, USA
* Corresponding author.
E-mail address: abuelmk@ccf.org

practical application of the procedure was only feasible after the 1989 advent of tacrolimus.[4] Despite waves of enthusiasm and disappointment, the continual evolution of the procedure was achievable as a result of continuous interplay between new advances in surgical techniques, immunosuppressive strategies, and postoperative management.[2,5]

Establishment of the current distinctive nomenclature has largely stemmed from the anatomic and surgical principles described with the original multivisceral transplant operation.[6–8] Elucidation of the mechanisms of allograft acceptance, along with the availability of new immunosuppressive agents, has been behind the introduction of novel immunosuppressive, immunomodulatory, and preconditioning strategies.[9,10] The cumulative increase in clinical experience with advances in molecular diagnostic techniques and the availability of new antimicrobial agents enhanced postoperative care.[1]

In 2000, the Centers for Medicare and Medicaid Services qualified intestinal and multivisceral transplantation as the standard of care for patients with irreversible gut failure who no longer can be maintained on parenteral nutrition (PN).[11] With the subsequent increase in worldwide experience, practical guidelines, including expansion of the initial indications, have evolved in recent years.[12] Despite the continual improvement in outcome, the procedure is still limited to patients with nutritional failure who no longer can be maintained on PN. In addition, most health care providers also mandate failure of gut rehabilitative efforts as a prerequisite for transplantation. However, it is imperative to emphasize that early transplantation, at centers of excellence, has been associated with many therapeutic advantages, including better survival with successful restoration of nutritional autonomy and quality of life.[5] Furthermore, halting the PN-associated native liver damage with early transplantation optimizes the deceased donor liver utilization for patients with isolated hepatic failure.

HISTORICAL EVOLUTION

Traced back to the pioneer experimental work of the 1912 Nobel Prize winner Alexis Carrel,[13] the modern history of multivisceral transplantation was assigned by the innovative experimental work and initial clinical attempts of Thomas Starzl.[14,15] In 1983, 20 years after his first successful canine multivisceral transplant, Starzl performed the first 2 multivisceral transplantations in humans with en bloc inclusion of the stomach, duodenum, pancreas, intestine, colon, and liver.[16] Both cases were children with gut and liver failure associated with short bowel syndrome, which were transplanted under cyclosporine-based immunosuppression. Although the first case died perioperatively from multisystem organ failure, the second multivisceral recipient survived more than 6 months with a fully functioning graft only to die from progressive post-transplant lymphoproliferative disease (PTLD).

In 1990, Grant and colleagues[17] published the first successful case of a lesser composite visceral allograft in humans. The combined liver-intestinal allograft was transplanted under cyclosporine-based immunosuppression using the simultaneously transplanted donor liver as an immunoprotective shield to the transplanted intestine. The replaced native liver had normal structural and synthetic functions but with antithrombin III deficiency. Ironically, FK-506, currently known as tacrolimus, was introduced in the same year by the Pittsburgh team, allowing the successful clinical transplantation of the intestine-only allograft without the need for simultaneous hepatic replacement.[18] These successful initial efforts created a wave of enthusiasm that increased the clinical feasibility and practicality of the different types of visceral transplantation. In addition, new modifications were introduced to both the donor and recipient transplant procedures.[5,11,19,20]

Full details of the historical evolution of immunosuppression and postoperative care are beyond the scope of this article.[1,3] In brief, the clinical introduction of interleukin (IL)-2 receptor antibodies and the different antilymphocyte preparations have contributed significantly to the evolution of the immunosuppressive regimen. Meanwhile, new insights into the mechanism of allograft acceptance and transplant tolerance have guided the effective utilization of these agents for induction therapy and recipient or donor pretreatment.[1] Advances in postoperative care were the result of cumulative experience, introduction of new diagnostic and biologic tools, and availability of effective antimicrobial agents.[5]

NOMENCLATURE

In 1991, the many faces of multivisceral and composite visceral transplantation were eloquently described and illustrated by Starzl and colleagues.[7] In essence, the intestine is the central core of any visceral allograft and the nomenclature is based on the type and number of the organs that are transplanted en bloc with the intestine (**Fig. 1**).[8,21] Accordingly, the cluster operation that entails en bloc replacement of the liver, pancreas, duodenum, and small portion of jejunum, with or without the stomach (**Fig. 2**) is commonly misnamed as a multivisceral transplantation. It is also imperative to differentiate between the terms multiorgan transplantation and multivisceral transplantation. The term multiorgan transplantation is defined as simultaneous or sequential individual organ transplantation without inclusion of the intestine. The term multivisceral transplantation is defined as en bloc implantation of the abdominal visceral organs, including the stomach and intestine.[22]

Composite visceral transplantation is a broader term encompassing multivisceral transplantation and any other combination of the visceral allograft with en bloc inclusion of the liver and/or pancreas (see **Fig. 1**). The multivisceral transplantation can be full or modified, including the stomach, duodenum, pancreas, and intestine, with or without the liver, respectively (see **Fig. 1**). The other composite visceral allografts

Intestine-Pancreas	Liver-Intestine[a]	Multivisceral	
		Full	Modified
		Stomach + Duodenum + Pancreas + Intestine + Liver	Stomach + Duodenum + Pancreas + Intestine
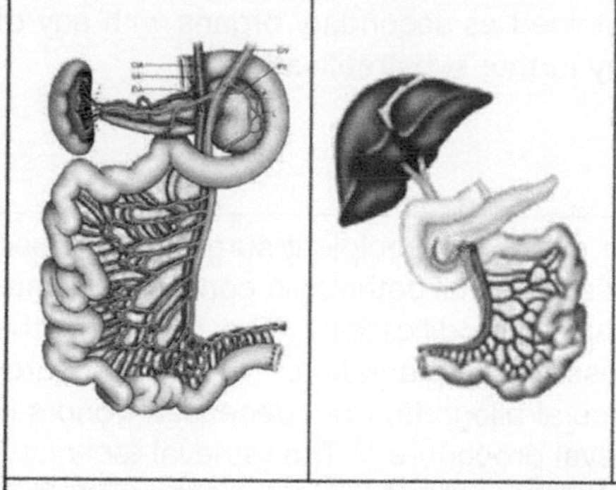		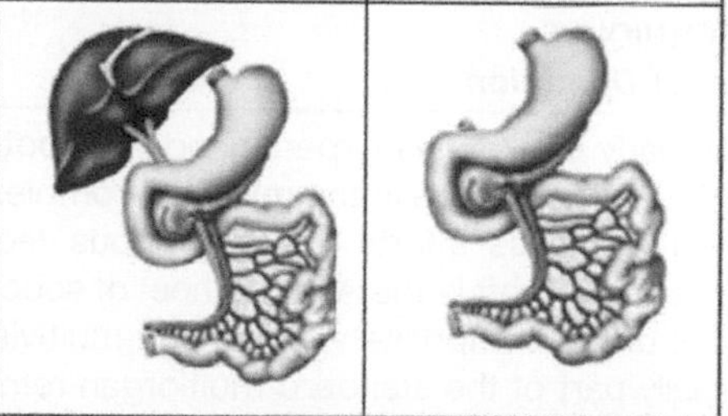	
		Descriptive	
• En bloc with colon and/or kidney	• En bloc with colon and/or kidney	• En bloc with colon and/or kidney • With preserved pancreaticoduodenal complex and/or spleen	

Fig. 1. Types of composite visceral allografts. [a] Inclusion of the pancreaticoduodenal complex is optional and commonly used for technical reasons. (*Reprinted by* permission from Springer Nature. Adapted from Fujiki M, Hashimoto H, Khanna A, et al. Technical innovation and visceral transplantation. In: Subramaniam K, Sakai T, editors. Anesthesia and perioperative care for organ transplantation. New York: Springer; 2017. p. 498.)

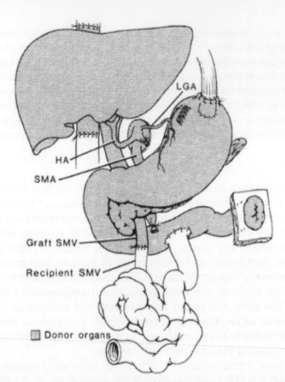

Fig. 2. Cluster graft, including stomach. HA, hepatic artery; LGA, left gastric artery; SMA, superior mesenteric artery; and SMV, superior mesenteric vein. (*From* Starzl TE, Todo S, Tzakis A, et al. The many faces of multivisceral transplantation. Surg Gynecol Obstet 1991;172(5):335-344. Reprinted with permission from the Journal of the American College of Surgeons, formerly Surgery Gynecology & Obstetrics.)

include the intestine and pancreas, with or without the liver (see **Fig. 1**). The donor colon, spleen, and/or kidney can always be retained as secondary organs with any of these allograft types without the need for any further substratification.[21]

TECHNIQUES
Donor Operation

The early challenges experienced with both donor and recipient surgery combined with organ shortage in the milieu of complex abdominal pathologic conditions stimulated relentless efforts toward various technical modifications. The quality of the visceral allograft is the Achilles heel of successful transplantation.[23] In brief, procurement of the composite visceral and multivisceral allografts from deceased donors is usually part of the standard multiorgan retrieval procedure.[11] The retrieval technique is based on the embryology and vascular blood supply of the gut organs (**Fig. 3**).[24] In recent years, Benedetti and colleagues introduced the living donor composite visceral transplantation with separate segmental liver and intestine.[25] It is fundamental for both deceased and live donor allografts to obtain good quality arterial and venous-free vascular grafts for the back table and in situ vascular reconstruction.

Recipient Surgery

The recipient operation with implantation of the different composite visceral allografts is often complex and technically challenging (**Fig. 4**).[26] The extent of abdominal

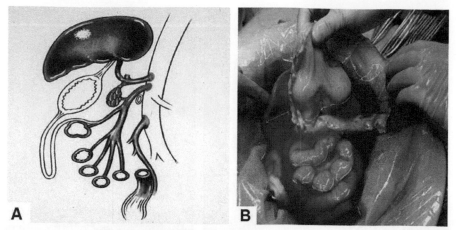

Fig. 3. (*A*) The embryonic anatomy of the foregut, midgut, and hindgut. (*B*) A multivisceral graft, including the stomach, duodenum, pancreas, liver, and intestine, in the ice cold organ preservation solution. Note that the spleen was used to handle the organs and was removed as part of the back table procedure. (*Courtesy of* Kareem Abu-Elmagd, MD, Cleveland, OH.)

dissection in patients who require a multivisceral transplantation is illustrated in **Fig. 5.** In selected patients with infected abdomen or extensive mesenteric desmoid tumor, an initial exploratory laparotomy is required as a first-stage operation to rescue candidacy for transplantation.[27,28] In the presence of limited central venous access, perioperative establishment of a reliable wide-bore venous access is required for prompt intraoperative resuscitation. Patients with multiple prior abdominal surgeries and organ failure often undergo careful major abdominal dissection with creation of a new abdominal domain. In addition, the extent of the abdominal evisceration procedure is modified according to the indications for transplantation, particularly in patients

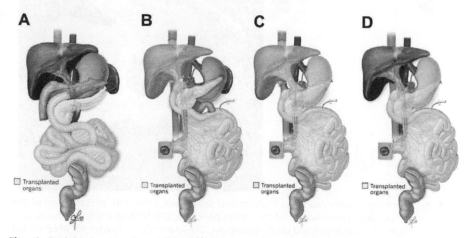

Fig. 4. Recipient operation; the different composite visceral allografts. (*A*) Intestine-pancreas. (*B*) Combined liver-intestine with en bloc pancreaticoduodenal complex. (*C*) Full multivisceral. (*D*) Modified multivisceral. (*Reprinted with* permission, Cleveland Clinic Center for Medical Art & Photography © 2005–2018. All Rights Reserved.)

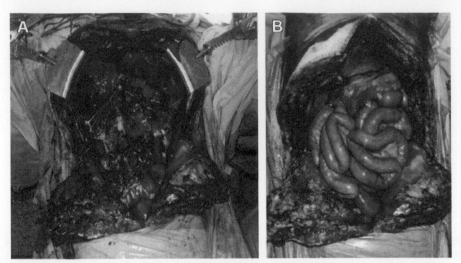

Fig. 5. Multivisceral transplantation. (*A*) Removal of diseased organs. (*B*) Reperfusion of new organs.

with gut dysmotility and Gardner syndrome.[20] When technically feasible, the native pancreaticoduodenal complex or the splenic compartment is preserved in those who are in need of full and modified multivisceral transplantation with merit to reduce risk of infection, PTLD, and diabetes (**Fig. 6**).[19,20,29]

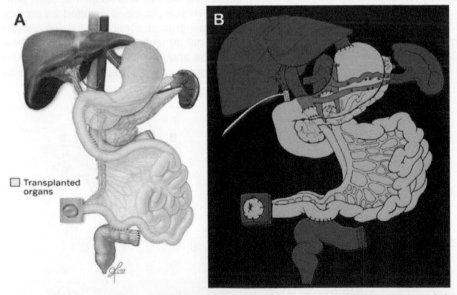

Fig. 6. Recipient operation; modified multivisceral transplantation with preservation of the native spleen. (*A*) With preservation of the native pancreas. (*B*) With inclusion of pancreas in the donor allograft. ((*A*) *Reprinted with permission,* Cleveland Clinic Center for Medical Art & Photography © 2005–2018. All Rights Reserved; and (*B*) *From* Abu-Elmagd K, Khanna A, Fujiki M, et al. Surgery for gut failure: Auto-reconstruction and allo-transplantation. In: Fazio V, Church JM, Delaney CP, Kiran RP, eds. Current Therapy in Colon and Rectal Surgery. Philadelphia, PA: Elsevier, Inc.; 2017. p. 379; with permission.)

The vascular reconstruction is technically demanding using back table and in situ techniques. The back table arterial reconstruction is required to establish a single or bifurcated arterial conduit for the allograft celiac and superior mesenteric arteries. A segment of the donor descending aorta is used for the single conduit, applying the Carrel-patch technique (**Fig. 7**). The donor common iliac artery with its external and internal arterial branches can be used for the bifurcated arterial conduit, particularly for the combined intestinal and pancreas composite visceral allograft (see **Fig. 1**).

In preparation for visceral allograft implantation, a free arterial graft using another segment of the donor descending thoracic aorta is placed on the infrarenal and, less frequently, the supraceliac native aorta (**Fig. 8**). Such a technique was introduced by the senior author to ensure an easy and safe vascular reconstruction before bringing the voluminous allograft into the operative field.[30] An interposition vein graft with proper orientation is also often needed to restore the venous drainage of the modified multivisceral and combined intestine-pancreas composite graft (see **Fig. 8**). The free common iliac donor vein graft is commonly placed on 1 of the recipient's major portal tributaries or the infrarenal vena cava. In patients who are in need of simultaneous liver replacement (liver-intestine or full multivisceral) with preservation of the native left upper quadrant organs, a permanent native portocaval shunt is created before or immediately after completion of the native hepatectomy (**Fig. 9**).

Visceral allograft implantation is initiated by the in vivo vascular reconstruction of both the arterial inflow and venous outflow of the en bloc contained organs (see **Fig. 4**). With liver-free composite allografts, including the intestine-duodenum-pancreas (combined intestine-pancreas) and stomach-duodenum-pancreas-

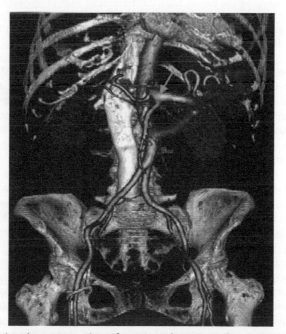

Fig. 7. A 3-dimensional reconstruction of computed tomography angiogram in a multivisceral recipient. Note the Carrel-patch reconstruction (*arrow*) that was performed on the back table containing both the celiac and superior mesenteric origin.

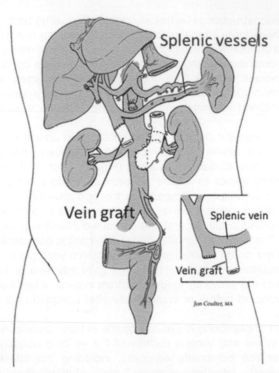

Fig. 8. Placement of interposition arterial and venous grafts on the native infrarenal aorta and the remnant stump of the native superior mesenteric vein or splenic vein, respectively. (*From* Cruz RJ, Costa G, Bond G, et al. Modified "liver-sparing" multivisceral transplant with preserved native spleen, pancreas, and duodenum: technique and long-term outcome. J Gastrointest Surg 2010;14:1714; with permission.)

intestine (modified multivisceral), the bifurcated or Carrel-patch arterial conduit is anastomosed to the placed infrarenal aortic or common iliac free arterial vascular graft. The venous reconstruction is guided by the allograft type. With simultaneous hepatic replacement, the venous drainage is established by anastomosing the donor suprahepatic cava to the main confluence of the native hepatic veins because most of these patients undergo hepatectomy using the piggyback technique (see **Fig. 4**B, C). With liver-free visceral transplantation, the bifurcated vein graft (intestine-pancreas) or the retained main portal vein stump (modified multivisceral) is anastomosed to the interposition vein graft that is commonly placed on the recipient portal vein or 1 of its main tributaries (see **Fig. 8**). In a few of these liver-free allograft recipients, the venous drainage is established into the native infrarenal inferior vena cava, particularly in those with hepatic parenchymal changes and mild elevation of the portal venous pressure.[31]

The gastrointestinal reconstruction is commonly dictated by the surgical anatomy of the retained native gut organs and type of visceral allograft. Foregut reconstruction is part of the full or modified multivisceral transplantation. The residual native stomach or abdominal esophagus is anastomosed to the anterior wall of the allograft stomach with pyloroplasty or pyloromyotomy performed as a drainage procedure (see **Fig. 4**C, D). In recipients of liver-intestinal allografts and those with preserved pancreaticoduodenal complex, midgut reconstruction is required to restore continuity between the native and transplanted gut. With liver-intestinal transplant, the very

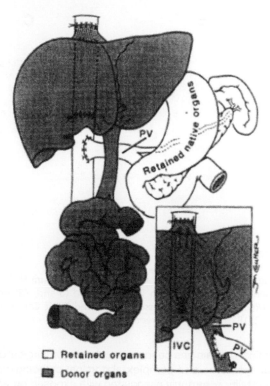

□ Retained organs

▨ Donor organs

Fig. 9. Drainage of the venous outflow of the retained native viscera in liver-intestinal recipients into their inferior vena cava (IVC) by portocaval shunt. PV, portal vein. *(From* Starzl TE, Todo S, Tzakis A, et al. The many faces of multivisceral transplantation. Surg Gynecol Obstet 1991;172(5):335-344. *Reprinted with permission from* the Journal of the American College of Surgeons, formerly Surgery Gynecology & Obstetrics.)

proximal allograft jejunum is anastomosed to the retained short segment of the native jejunum in end-to-end, end-to-side, or side-to-side fashion (**Fig. 10**). With retained native duodenum, a piggyback duodenoduodenal reconstruction is performed (see **Figs. 4**A and **6**A).

Hindgut reconstruction is commonly performed in recipients with residual colon or rectum, with creation of a diverting chimney (**Fig. 11**A) or simple loop ileostomy (**Fig. 11**B) to facilitate surveillance biopsies. In patients with pseudoobstruction, a hindgut reconstruction is still performed with total abdominal colectomy and creation of an ileosigmoid anastomosis. Patients with previous proctocolectomy who are not candidates for a pull-through operation receive a permanent allograft end ileostomy (**Fig. 11**C). Surgical closure of the temporary vents is generally performed within 6 months of transplantation, guided by the postoperative course and functional recovery of the visceral graft.

In recent years, colonic conduits were used for foregut and hindgut reconstruction. An interposition segment of the native colon is used for foregut reconstruction to reduce the number of required allograft organs (**Fig. 12**A). The donor colon was also used en bloc with the visceral allograft to restore hindgut reconstruction and eliminate the need for lifelong end ileostomy (**Fig. 12**B).With technical details described elsewhere, inclusion of the donor colon in the visceral graft improves functional outcome and quality of life when it is clinically indicated.[32]

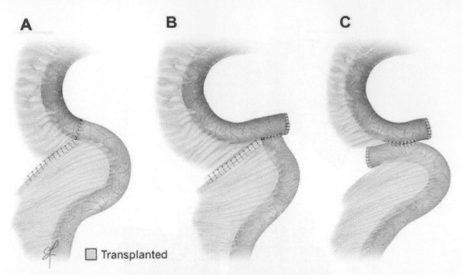

Fig. 10. Gastrointestinal reconstruction. Proximal allograft jejunum is anastomosed to the retained short segment of native jejunum in an (*A*) end-to-end, (*B*) end-to-side, or (*C*) side-to-side fashion. (*Reprinted with permission*, Cleveland Clinic Center for Medical Art & Photography © 2005–2018. All Rights Reserved.)

Loss of the abdominal domain has been among the major surgical challenges in patients with short gut syndrome and complex abdominal pathologic conditions. With the morbidity and mortality commonly associated with exposed organs, several innovative surgical tactics have been introduced, including implantation of tissue expanders before transplant, use of small-for-size allografts, visceral allograft reduction, component separation techniques, myocutaneous flaps, acellular dermal allograft, synthetic mesh, and simultaneous vascularized abdominal wall or nonvascularized rectus fascia transplant.[33–37] Nonetheless, it has been the authors' experience that small-for-size allografts and judicious intraoperative fluid resuscitation allows successful primary skin closure in most recipients, without the need for immediate major abdominal wall reconstructive procedures.[28]

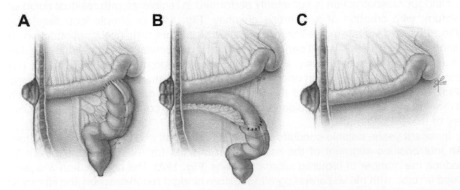

Fig. 11. Hindgut reconstruction with creation of a (*A*) chimney ileostomy, (*B*) simple loop ileostomy, or (*C*) end ileostomy. (*Reprinted with permission*, Cleveland Clinic Center for Medical Art & Photography © 2005–2018. All Rights Reserved.)

A   B

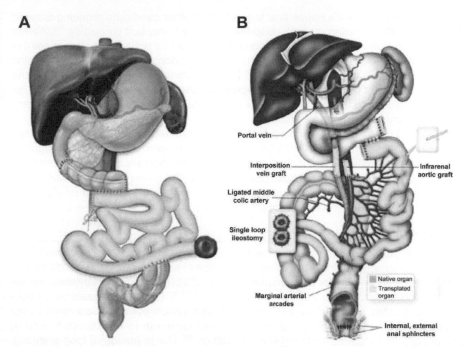

Portal vein

Interposition vein graft

Ligated middle colic artery

Single loop ileostomy

Marginal arterial arcades

Infrarenal aortic graft

Native organ
Transplanted organ

Internal, external anal sphincters

Fig. 12. (A) Foregut reconstruction with interposition segment of the native colon. (B) Hindgut pull-through reconstruction with en bloc colon and intestinal transplantation. ([A] *Reprinted with permission*, Cleveland Clinic Center for Medical Art & Photography © 2005-2018. All Rights Reserved; and [B] *From* Hashimoto K, Costa G, Khanna A, Fujiki M, Quintini C, Abu-Elmagd K. Recent advances in intestinal and multivisceral transplantation. Adv Surg 2015;45:31–63.)

CURRENT CLINICAL PRACTICE
Indications

Visceral transplantation with different organ combinations has been successfully used for patients with gut failure due to a wide spectrum of structural and functional gastrointestinal disorders.[11,38] It is also indicated for patients with complex abdominal pathologic conditions. According to the international Intestinal Transplant Registry and extensive single-center experience, the leading indication for visceral transplantation is short gut syndrome due to mesenteric ischemia, end-stage Crohn's disease in adults, and congenital disorders in the pediatric population.[5,38] Other common indications include global gut dysmotility, neoplastic disorders, and primary or secondary enterocyte dysfunction. Diffuse portomesenteric venous thrombosis and bariatric surgery-associated gut failure have recently emerged as infrequent indications for gut transplantation.[26]

Diffuse gastrointestinal disorders commonly dictate the need for multivisceral replacement with inclusion of the liver in those with concomitant liver failure and extensive portomesenteric venous thrombosis. Simultaneous replacement of the native liver without advanced cirrhosis or overt hepatic failure should not be entertained solely because of the biological privilege of the simultaneously transplanted liver.[5] However, replacement of a fully functioning native liver could be justified in selected patients with recurrent chronic rejection of an isolated intestinal allograft. As previously described, the recipient's native liver is given to another candidate requiring isolated liver transplantation using the well-described domino transplant procedure.[5] Different modalities of multivisceral transplantation are also used for patients who are in need of retransplantation, particularly those with a hostile abdomen. The combined en bloc intestine-pancreas transplant is required for patients with irreversible intestinal and beta cell failure. In patients with end-stage renal disease, the donor kidney is transplanted en bloc with the liver-intestine or multivisceral, and separately with the combined intestine-pancreas transplant.

In contrast to isolated intestinal transplantation, the need for or failure of PN therapy is not an essential prerequisite for some of the liver-free composite visceral allografts. In most of these patients, the indications for transplantation are commonly life-saving because of premalignant and diffuse gut disorders in the milieu of complex abdominal pathologic conditions. This is compounded by the lack of effective gut rehabilitation modalities for these complex patients.[27]

Contraindications

Significant cardiopulmonary insufficiency, incurable malignancy, persistent life-threatening intraabdominal or systemic infections, and severe immune deficiency syndromes with inability for pretransplant successful stem cell transplantation are absolute contraindications to visceral transplantation.[11,26] Lack of adequate social support has recently emerged as a relative contraindication owing to associated poor long-term survival. Accordingly, all efforts should be made to reestablish functional social support before considering transplantation.[39] The presence of long-standing, controlled neuropsychiatric disorders should not preclude transplantation as successful rehabilitation because visceral transplantation has recently been documented in both children and adults.[39] Similarly, history of gut malignancy, loss of central venous access, and older age should not be solely considered as a contraindication for transplantation.

Evaluation

All patients undergo a thorough evaluation process to assess extent of gut failure, candidacy for transplantation, type of required allograft, and presence of contraindications for transplantation. The assessment includes clinical, biochemical, radiologic, endoscopic, and histologic studies. Equally important is the thorough socioeconomic and psychiatric evaluation with the establishment of management tactics to address the underlying pathologic conditions and rescue candidacy for transplantation. Special attention should be paid to the absolute and relative transplant contraindications as previously discussed.

The cause of gut failure commonly dictates the need for special laboratory, endoscopic, and imaging studies. The innate and adaptive immune status should be evaluated in patients with hereditary or congenital disorders to assess the potential risk of graft-versus-host disease after transplantation. Pan endoscopy is performed in patients with hereditary neoplastic disorders to assess the extent of the dysplastic syndrome and coexistent malignancy. Central venous angiography of both upper and lower extremities is mandatory in patients with a history of central venous thrombosis to establish a reliable venous access plan at the time of transplant. Computerized tomography and/or standard abdominal visceral angiography is indicated for patients with history of portomesenteric venous thrombosis to assess candidacy for liver transplant alone, liver plus intestine with the technical feasibility of creating a native portocaval shunt, or multivisceral transplant with complete evisceration of the left upper quadrant abdominal organs with totally occluded splenic venous system. The surgical anatomy of the residual gastrointestinal tract, particularly of the hindgut, is radiologically and manometrically studied to assess potential candidacy for hindgut reconstruction or a pull-through operation.

Waiting List Management

The establishment of clinical guidelines for proper management of the composite and multivisceral candidates on the United Network of Organ Sharing (UNOS) waitlist has been comprehensively addressed elsewhere.[40] The complexity and dynamic nature of the clinical management of these challenging patients is emanating from the expected continual risk of PN-associated complications, including life-threatening infection, vanishing of central venous access, and progression of liver damage. Despite the periodic changes in the UNOS regulations and organ allocation, the log relative risk of mortality for liver-intestine continues to be 3-fold that of the liver-only candidates (**Fig. 13**).[40] Further development of central and portomesenteric venous thrombosis can potentially preclude or upgrade the type of required allograft, respectively. In contrast, recent advances in PN management have the potential to ameliorate cholestatic liver dysfunction and downgrade the type of required composite visceral graft with preservation of native liver.

Postoperative Care

Management of immunosuppression, monitoring of allograft function, and diagnosis with prompt treatment of recipient microbial infection are the 3 essential components of postoperative care. With the high immunogenicity of the gut allograft, concerted efforts have been made toward innovative immunosuppressive strategies.[27] One of the most important contributions has been the introduction of induction therapy and recipient preconditioning to the tacrolimus-based immunosuppression regimen.[1]

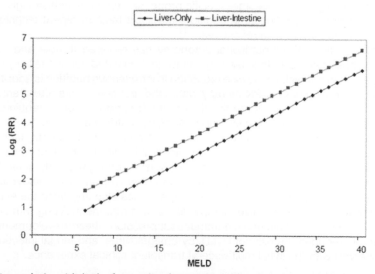

Fig. 13. Log relative risk (RR) of mortality for combined liver-intestine candidates compared with liver-only candidates on the Organ Procurement and Transplantation Network waiting list. (*From* Abu-Elmagd K. Intestinal and multivisceral transplant waiting list: clinical management according to allograft type and current organ allocation system. In: Kirk A, Knechtle S, Larsen C, editors. Textbook of organ transplantation. 1st edition. Oxford (United Kingdom): Wiley-Blackwell; 2014. p. 492; with permission.)

The commonly used pharmacologic and biologic agents are cyclophosphamide, anti-IL-2 receptor humanized antibodies, rabbit antithymocyte globulin (rATG), and alemtuzumab. In addition, azathioprine, mycophenolate mofetil, and mammalian target of rapamycin (mTOR) inhibitors have been used as an adjunct maintenance therapy. Immunomodulatory strategies, including donor pretreatment, bone marrow augmentation, and allograft irradiation, have also been used to improve the outcome with multivisceral transplantation.[1,31,38] Interestingly, there have been no efforts among all major centers to tailor the immunosuppressive regimen according to the type of the visceral allograft, with or without inclusion of the liver. It is the authors' recommendation that future prospective studies are required to address the efficacy of different immunosuppressive protocols designed based on the type of the visceral allograft, with special reference to the liver.

Monitoring of the recipient alloimmune response and allograft functions has been the central core of postoperative care. Monitoring of graft rejection is achieved by protocol ileoscopies with multiple random intestinal biopsies and serial measurement of circulating donor-specific antibodies (DSA).[31,41] The diagnosis of acute cellular, humoral, and chronic rejection is established according to previously defined histopathologic criteria.[42,43] The diagnosis of liver rejection is suspected in patients with transaminitis and confirmed by the histopathologic examination of a Tru-Cut liver biopsy. Rejection of the pancreatic allograft is suspected in patients with significant elevation of serum amylase and lipase, without evident causes of nonimmunologic pancreatitis.

The dynamic process of graft-versus-host reaction with establishment of macrochimerism and microchimerism has been recently monitored by the serial detection of circulating donor cells in the recipient peripheral blood.[5] The diagnosis of graft-versus-host disease is confirmed by histopathologic and immunocytochemical studies that allow identification of donor leukocytes in the peripheral blood and targeted organs. The methodology includes polymerase chain reaction (PCR) techniques, in situ hybridization using Y-chromosome–specific probe, and the immunohistologic staining of donor-specific HLA antigens. In addition, the short tandem repeat technique has been more frequently used in recent years.[44]

The achievement of full nutritional autonomy has required flexible and complex management strategies. Enteric feeding is commonly initiated during the early postoperative period. In parallel, a stepwise reduction in intravenous nutrition is adopted with complete discontinuation of PN therapy within the first few weeks after transplantation. Temporary and intermittent reinstitution of PN support is often required in patients with severe allograft rejection and suboptimal nutritional status.

With cumulative clinical experience, advanced molecular diagnostic techniques, and new antimicrobial drugs, the outcome after multivisceral transplantation has substantially improved.[5] The availability of the PCR assay prompted early detection and serial monitoring of peripheral blood viremia with Epstein-Barr virus and cytomegalovirus. The introduction of new antimicrobial agents has also improved the efficacy of infection prophylaxis, preemptive therapy, and active treatment. Along with stepwise judicious reduction in maintenance immunosuppression, these developments have considerably reduced the risks of PTLD, cytomegalovirus, and fungal infections that were observed with the initial multivisceral transplant clinical experience.[5]

LONG-TERM OUTCOME

The growing global experience with visceral transplantation is a testimony of the continual improvement in the procedure's short-term and long-term efficacy over the last 3 decades. Such an achievement is a result of innovative surgical techniques, novel immunosuppressive protocols, and better postoperative management. The current results justify the recent elevation of the procedure level to that of other abdominal organs, with the privilege to permanently reside in a respected place in the surgical armamentarium.

Survival

The worldwide and largest single-center cumulative experience has repeatedly demonstrated steady improvement in 1-year and 5-year actuarial patient and allograft survival, with current rates comparable to pancreas and lung allografts (**Fig. 14**).[5,27,38] Beyond the 5-year milestone, the longest and largest single-center series documented a 10-year patient survival of 75% and 60% at 15 years with a respective graft survival of 59% and 50%.[39] Loss of graft function and complications of immunosuppression continue to be the major threat to long-term survival, with rejection, infection, and renal failure being the leading causes of death. Interestingly, the cumulative risk of infection has been significantly higher among the multivisceral recipients compared with other visceral allograft patients (**Fig. 15A**).[5] Meanwhile, the liver-free visceral allografts experienced a significantly higher risk of cumulative graft loss due to rejection (**Fig. 15B**).[5]

Several predictors of survival outcome for both patient and allograft have been recently published.[39] The lack of social support and absence of the liver as part of the composite and multivisceral grafts have emerged as highly significant risk factors for patient and graft survival, respectively (**Table 1**).[39] The immunoprotective effect of the liver can be potentially explained in the context of ameliorating the detrimental effect of DSA on the visceral allograft survival (**Fig. 16**).[41] Other important risk factors include early rejection, recipient sex and age, splenectomy, retransplantation, HLA mismatch, and type of immunosuppression, with variable weight of statistical significance.[5,39]

Graft Function

The ability to restore nutritional autonomy is the second most important indicator of successful visceral transplantation. A high rate of freedom from intravenous nutrition

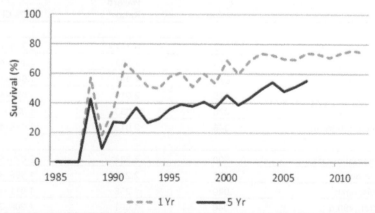

Fig. 14. A times series analysis of the 1-year and 5-year actuarial graft survival shows significant improvement over time (*P*<.001). (*From* Grant D, Abu-Elmagd K, Mazariegos G, et al. Intestinal transplant registry report: global activity and trends. Am J Transplant 2015;15:214; with permission.)

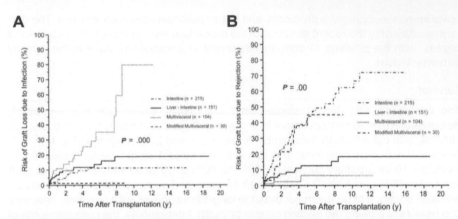

Fig. 15. Cumulative risk of graft loss due to (*A*) infection and (*B*) acute and chronic rejection according to type of visceral allograft. (*From* Abu-Elmagd KM, Costa G, Bond G, et al. Five hundred intestinal and multivisceral transplantations at a single center: major advances with new challenges. Ann Surg 2009;250:576; with permission.)

with maintained nutritional status and significant improvement in body mass index has been documented in the literature (**Fig. 17**).[38,39] The adult recipients maintain normal serum albumin and trace elements with improved skeletal health (**Fig. 18**).[39] Most children experience fairly normal linear growth, with a few requiring hormonal replacement.

The failure to achieve full nutritional autonomy in a few of the composite and multivisceral recipients is mainly due to persistent allograft dysmotility and steatorrhea resulting from allograft denervation and lymphatic disruption inherent to the transplant procedure. With the clinical availability of normothermic ex vivo perfusion technology, the unwanted effect of ischemia reperfusion could be ameliorated.[45] It is also

Table 1 Long-term survival risk factors for visceral transplant			
Risk Factor	**P Value**	**Hazard Ratio**	**95% CI**
Patient			
Lack of social support	.000	6.132	3.370–11.160
Rejection <90 d	.016	2.363	1.172–4.765
Female recipient	.025	1.992	1.089–3.646
Recipient age >20 y	.025	2.014	1.093–3.711
Retransplantation	.026	2.053	1.089–3.873
No preconditioning	.046	2.013	1.013–4.997
Graft			
Liver-free allograft	.000	3.224	2.026–5.132
Splenectomy	.001	2.212	1.396–3.506
HLA mismatch	.040	1.258	1.011–1.565
Rejection <90 d	.046	1.601	1.008–2.541
PTLD	.085	1.638	0.934–2.872

From Abu-Elmagd K. The concept of gut rehabilitation and the future of visceral transplantation. Nat Rev Gastroenterol Hepatol 2015;12:114; with permission.

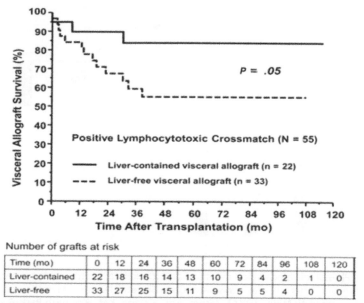

Fig. 16. The immunoprotective effect of the liver has been recently explained by ameliorating the detrimental effect of DSA on the visceral allograft survival. (*From* Abu-Elmagd KM, Wu G, Costa G, et al. Preformed and de novo donor specific antibodies in visceral transplantation: long-term outcome with special reference to the liver. Am J Transplant 2012;12:3054; with permission.)

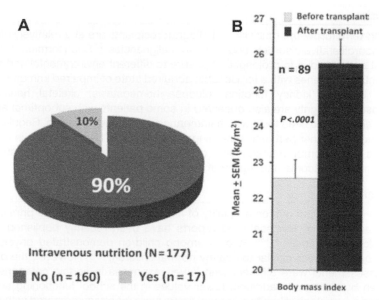

Fig. 17. Nutritional autonomy after visceral transplantation. (*A*) Achievement of enteric autonomy defined by freedom from intravenous nutrition and fluid supplement. (*B*) Body mass index before and after transplantation. (*From* Abu-Elmagd KM, Kosmach-Park B, Costa G, et al. Long-term survival, nutritional autonomy, and quality of life after intestinal and multivisceral transplantation. Ann Surg 2012;256:499; with permission.)

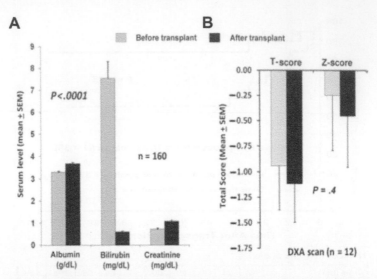

Fig. 18. (*A*) Physiologic biochemical measures and (*B*) skeletal health in a large single-center series before and after visceral transplantation. Skeletal health was measured by dual-energy x-ray absorptiometry (DXA). (*From* Abu-Elmagd KM, Kosmach-Park B, Costa G, et al. Long-term survival, nutritional autonomy, and quality of life after intestinal and multivisceral transplantation. Ann Surg 2012;256:500; with permission.)

reasonable to think that the altered allograft microbiota may play a significant role in allograft dysfunction and recipient wellbeing.

Morbidities

With long-term follow-up, multivisceral allograft recipients are at a relatively high risk of lymphoproliferative disorders and de novo malignancies.[39] Such formidable threats are most probably due to prolonged exposure to different environmental and nonenvironmental oncogenes with a foreseeable acquired state of impaired immune surveillance.[46] Impaired kidney function, glucose homeostasis, skeletal health, and cardiovascular integrity are also observed in some patients with suboptimal allograft function and chronic need for heavy maintenance immunosuppression. Regular tumor surveillance and other pertinent screening protocols have been effective in the early diagnosis and prompt management of these unique recipients, with sustained improvement in outcome and quality of life.[39]

Quality of Life

With improved survival outcome, quality of life has become among the primary therapeutic endpoints. A few scattered reports have been recently published among both children and adults.[47–58] Studies among children demonstrated physical and psychosocial functions similar to healthy normal children.[47,48] However, the parental proxy assessments were different with lower responses in certain categories than that given by children. In addition, lower values in the school functioning subcategories and psychological health summary score were reported compared with healthy children.[48] In adults, most published studies on health-related quality of life have demonstrated improvement in many of the domains, with better rehabilitative indices than PN.[39] Except for depression, successful transplantation offsets the deprived effect of both PN and disease gravity in most domains (**Fig. 19**).[39]

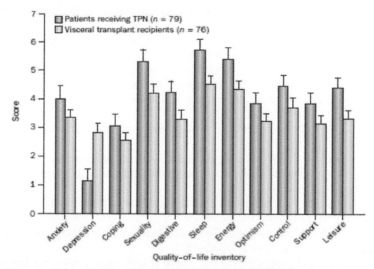

Fig. 19. Reversal of the depressed effect of total parenteral nutrition (TPN) on most quality of life domains, except depression, after visceral transplantation. (*From* Abu-Elmagd K. The concept of gut rehabilitation and the future of visceral transplantation. Nat Rev Gastroenterol Hepatol 2015;12:115; with permission.)

The socioeconomic milestones have also been used to assess the rehabilitative efficacy of visceral transplantation in all age groups.[39] A high education score was reported with sustained cognitive, psychosocial, and physical functions. In addition, the ability to create a nuclear family, along with high Lansky and Karnofsky performance scores, are demonstrated and comprehensively reported.[39] The data have also been in favor of early consideration for visceral transplantation to further improve quality of life by reducing the risk of organic brain-dysfunction–related morbidities associated with brain atrophy, cerebral vascular insufficiency, micronutrient deficiencies, trace element toxicities, and liver-failure.[59–62] Accordingly, early consideration of transplantation is strongly recommended for patients with irreversible gut failure who are not suitable candidates for autologous gut rehabilitation.

SUMMARY

Composite visceral and multivisceral transplantation continues to evolve as a lifesaving therapy for patients with irreversible metabolic, parenchymal, and functional gut failure. The procedure has also been used to rescue patients with complex abdominal pathologic conditions that are not amenable to current conventional medical and surgical modalities. Despite all efforts, the field continues to face the challenges of immunologic monitoring and longevity of the liver-free visceral allografts. With new insights into the biology of gut immunity and mechanisms of transplant acceptance, the establishment of less complex postoperative care and the achievement of a drug-free allograft acceptance are within reach.

REFERENCES

1. Abu-Elmagd KM, Costa G, Bond GJ, et al. Evolution of the immunosuppressive strategies for the intestinal and multivisceral recipients with special reference to

allograft immunity and achievement of partial tolerance. Transpl Int 2009;22: 96–109.

2. Grant D, Abu-Elmagd K, Reyes J, et al. 2003 report of the intestine transplant registry: a new era has dawned. Ann Surg 2005;241:607–13.

3. Nassar A, Fujiki M, Khanna A, et al. The historic evolution of intestinal and multivisceral transplantation. In: Subramaniam K, Sakai T, editors. Anesthesia and perioperative care for organ transplantation. New York: Springer Science+Business Media LLC; 2017. p. 487–96.

4. Starzl TE. FK 506 for human liver, kidney, and pancreas transplantation. Lancet 1989;2:1000–4.

5. Abu-Elmagd KM, Costa G, Bond G, et al. Five hundred intestinal and multivisceral transplantations at a single center: major advances with new challenges. Ann Surg 2009;250:567–81.

6. Starzl TE, Kaupp HA Jr. Mass homotransplantations of abdominal organs in dogs. Surg Forum 1960;11:28–30.

7. Starzl TE, Todo S, Tzakis A, et al. The many faces of multivisceral transplantation. Surg Gynecol Obstet 1991;172:335–44.

8. Abu-Elmagd KM. Preservation of the native spleen, duodenum, and pancreas in patients with multivisceral transplantation: nomenclature, dispute of origin, and proof of premise. Transplantation 2007;84:1208–9.

9. Starzl TE, Demetris AJ, Trucco M, et al. Cell migration and chimerism after whole-organ transplantation: the basic graft acceptance. Hepatology 1993;17:1127–52.

10. Starzl TE, Zinkernagel RM. Transplantation tolerance from a historical perspective. Nat Rev Immunol 2001;1:233–9.

11. Abu-Elmagd K, Bond G, Reyes J, et al. Intestinal transplantation: a coming of age. Adv Surg 2002;36:65–101.

12. Abu-Elmagd K. Intestinal transplantation: indications and patient selection. In: Langnas AN, Goulet O, Quigley EM, et al, editors. Intestinal failure: diagnosis, management and transplantation. Malden, Massachusetts: Blackwell Publishing; 2008. p. 245–53.

13. Carrel A. La technique operatoire des anastmoses vaculaires et la transplantation des visceres. Lyon MEO 1902;98:859–64.

14. Starzl TE, Kaupp HA Jr, Brock DR, et al. Homotransplantation of multiple visceral organs. Am J Surg 1962;103:219–29.

15. Starzl TE, Miller C, Bronznik B, et al. An improved technique for multiple organ harvesting. Surg Gynecol Obstet 1987;165:343–8.

16. Starzl TE, Rowe MI, Todo S, et al. Transplantation of multiple abdominal viscera. JAMA 1989;261:1449–57.

17. Grant D, Wall W, Mimeault R, et al. Successful small-bowel/liver transplantation. Lancet 1990;335:181–4.

18. Todo S, Tzakis AG, Abu-Elmagd K, et al. Intestinal transplantation in composite visceral grafts or alone. Ann Surg 1992;216:223–34.

19. Cruz RJ, Costa G, Bond G, et al. Modified "liver-sparing" multivisceral transplant with preserved native spleen, pancreas, and duodenum: technique and long-term outcome. J Gastrointest Surg 2010;14:1709–21.

20. Cruz RJ, Costa G, Bond GJ, et al. Modified multivisceral transplantation with spleen-preserving pancreaticoduodenectomy for patients with familial adenomatous polyposis "Gardner's syndrome". Transplantation 2011;91:1417–23.

21. Fujiki M, Hashimoto H, Khanna A, et al. Technical innovation and visceral transplantation. In: Subramaniam K, Sakai T, editors. Anesthesia and perioperative care for organ transplantation. New York: Springer; 2017. p. 497–511.

22. Abu-Elmagd KM. The small bowel contained allografts: existing and proposed nomenclature. Am J Transplant 2011;11:184–5.
23. Nickkholgh A, Contin P, Abu-Elmagd K, et al. Intestinal transplantation: review of operative techniques. Clin Transpl 2013;27:56–65.
24. Abu-Elmagd K, Reyes J, Fung JJ. Clinical intestinal transplantation: recent advances and future consideration. In: Norman DJ, Turka LA, editors. Primer on transplantation. 2nd edition. Mt Laurel (NJ): American Society of Transplantation; 2001. p. 610–25.
25. Garcia-Roca R, Tzvetanov IG, Jeon H, et al. Successful living donor intestinal transplantation in cross-match positive recipients: initial experience. World J Gastrointest Surg 2016;8:101–5.
26. Abu-Elmagd K, Khanna A, Fujiki M, et al. Surgery for gut failure: auto-reconstruction and allo-transplantation. In: Fazio V, Church JM, Delaney CP, et al, editors. Current therapy in colon and rectal surgery. Philadelphia: Elsevier, Inc; 2017. p. 372–84.
27. Abu-Elmagd K. The concept of gut rehabilitation and the future of visceral transplantation. Nat Rev Gastroenterol Hepatol 2015;12:108–20.
28. Hashimoto K, Costa G, Khanna A, et al. Recent advances in intestinal and multivisceral transplantation. Adv Surg 2015;49:31–63.
29. Abu-Elmagd K, Reyes J, Todo S, et al. Clinical intestinal transplantation: new perspectives and immunologic considerations. J Am Coll Surg 1998;186:512–27.
30. Abu-Elmagd K, Fung J, Bueno J, et al. Logistics and technique for procurement of intestinal, pancreatic and hepatic grafts from the same donor. Ann Surg 2000; 232:680–7.
31. Abu-Elmagd K, Reyes J, Bond G, et al. Clinical intestinal transplantation: a decade of experience at a single center. Ann Surg 2001;234:404–16.
32. Eid KR, Costa G, Bond GJ, et al. An innovative sphincter preserving pull-through technique with en bloc colon and small bowel transplantation. Am J Transplant 2010;10:1940–6.
33. Carlsen BT, Farmer DG, Busuttil RW, et al. Incidence and management of abdominal wall defects after intestinal and multivisceral transplantation. Plast Reconstr Surg 2007;119:1247–55.
34. Mangus RS, Kubal CA, Tector AJ, et al. Closure of the abdominal wall with acellular dermal allograft in intestinal transplantation. Am J Transplant 2012;12:S55–9.
35. Watson MJ, Kundu N, Coppa C, et al. Role of tissue expanders in patients with loss of abdominal domain awaiting intestinal transplantation. Transpl Int 2013; 26:1184–90.
36. Gondolesi G, Selvaggi G, Tzakis A, et al. Use of the abdominal rectus fascia as a nonvascularized allograft for abdominal wall closure after liver, intestinal, and multivisceral transplantation. Transplantation 2009;87:1884–8.
37. Levi DM, Tzakis AG, Kato T, et al. Transplantation of the abdominal wall. Lancet 2003;361:2173–6.
38. Grant D, Abu-Elmagd K, Masariegos G, et al. Intestinal transplant registry report: global activity and trends. Am J Transplant 2015;15:210–9.
39. Abu-Elmagd KM, Kosmach-Park B, Costa G, et al. Long-term survival, nutritional autonomy, and quality of life after intestinal and multivisceral transplantation. Ann Surg 2012;256:494–508.
40. Abu-Elmagd K. Intestinal and multivisceral transplant waiting list: clinical management according to allograft type and current organ allocation system. In: Kirk A, Knechtle S, Larsen C, editors. Textbook of organ transplantation. 1st edition. Oxford (United Kingdom): Wiley-Blackwell; 2014. p. 489–94.

41. Abu-Elmagd KM, Wu G, Costa G, et al. Preformed and de novo donor specific antibodies in visceral transplantation: long-term outcome with special reference to the liver. Am J Transplant 2012;12:3047–360.

42. Lee RG, Nakamura K, Tsamandas AC, et al. Pathology of human intestinal transplantation. Gastroenterology 1996;110:2009–12.

43. Wu T, Abu-Elmagd K, Bond G, et al. A clinicopathologic study of isolated intestinal allografts with preformed IgG lymphocytotoxic antibodies. Hum Pathol 2004; 35:1332–9.

44. Thiede C, Bornhauser M, Oelschlagel U, et al. Sequential monitoring of chimerism and detection of minimal residual disease after allogeneic blood stem cell transplantation (BSCT) using multiplex PCR amplification of short tandem repeat markers. Leukemia 2001;15:293–302.

45. Boehnert MU, Yeung JC, Bazerbachi F, et al. Normothermic acelluar ex vivo perfusion reduces liver and bile duct injury of pig livers retrieved after cardiac death. Am J Transplant 2013;13:1441–9.

46. Abu-Elmagd KM, Mazariegos G, Costa G, et al. Lymphoproliferative disorders and de novo malignancies in intestinal and multivisceral recipients: improved outcomes with new outlooks. Transplantation 2009;88:926–34.

47. Sudan D, Iyer K, Horslen S, et al. Assessment of quality of life after pediatric intestinal transplantation by parents and pediatric recipients using the child health questionnaire. Transplant Proc 2002;34:963–4.

48. Ngo KD, Farmer DG, McDiarmid SV, et al. Pediatric health-related quality of life after intestinal transplantation. Pediatr Transplant 2011;15:849–54.

49. DiMartini A, Rovera GM, Graham TO, et al. Quality of life after small intestinal transplantation and among home parenteral nutrition patients. JPEN J Parenter Enteral Nutr 1998;22:357–62.

50. Rovera GM, DiMartini A, Schoen RE, et al. Quality of life of patients after intestinal transplantation. Transplantation 1998;66:1141–5.

51. Rovera GM, DiMartini A, Graham TO, et al. Quality of life after intestinal transplantation and on total parenteral nutrition. Transplant Proc 1998;30:2513–4.

52. Stenn PG, Lammens P, Houle L, et al. Psychiatric psychosocial and ethical aspects of small bowel transplantation. Transplant Proc 1992;24:1251–2.

53. Cameron EA, Binnie JA, Jamieson NV, et al. Quality of life in adults following small bowel transplantation. Transplant Proc 2002;34:965–6.

54. Pironi L, Paganelli F, Lauro A, et al. Quality of life on home parenteral nutrition or after intestinal transplantation. Transplant Proc 2006;38:1673–5.

55. Sudan DL, Iverson A, Weseman RA, et al. Assessment of function, growth and development, and long-term quality of life after small bowel transplantation. Transplant Proc 2000;32:1211–2.

56. Golfieri L, Lauro A, Tossani E, et al. Psychological adaptation and quality of life of adult intestinal transplant recipients: University of Bologna experience. Transplant Proc 2010;42:42–4.

57. O'Keefe SJ, Emerling M, Koritsky D, et al. Nutrition and quality of life following small intestinal transplantation. Am J Gastroenterol 2007;102:1093–100.

58. Pironi L, Baxter JP, Lauro A, et al. Assessment of quality of life on home parenteral nutrition and after intestinal transplantation using treatment-specific questionnaires. Am J Transplant 2012;12:S60–6.

59. Idoate MA, Martinez AJ, Bueno J, et al. The neuropathology of intestinal failure and small bowel transplantation. Acta Neuropathol 1999;97:502–8.

60. Dekaban AS. Changes in brain weights during the span of human life: relation of brain weights to body heights and body weights. Ann Neurol 1978;4:345–56.

61. El-Tatawy S, Badrawi N, El Bishlawy A. Cerebral atrophy in infants with protein energy malnutrition. AJNR Am J Neuroradiol 1983;4:434–6.
62. Kawakubo K, Iida M, Matsumoto T, et al. Progressive encephalopathy in a Crohn's disease patient on long-term total parenteral nutrition: possible relationship to selenium deficiency. Postgrad Med J 1994;70:215–9.

Safe Living Following Solid Organ Transplantation

Barbra M. Blair, MD

KEYWORDS

- Solid organ transplantation • Vaccination • Food safety • Travel advice
- Infection prevention

KEY POINTS

- Infections after transplant can have significant impact on a patient's as well as their organ's survival. Several strategies can be used to minimize risk of acquisition of such infections.
- Vaccination against viral and bacterial illnesses, carefully timed preferably pretransplant, as well as safe living strategies posttransplant can afford protection against infections.
- Careful assessment pretransplant combined with a strategy of ongoing patient education pretransplant and posttransplant can assist patients with maintaining their health.

INTRODUCTION

Living safely after organ transplantation requires an integrated care continuum that starts before transplant and ideally even before the development of end organ disease. In order to minimize a solid organ transplant (SOT) recipient's risk for infection and risk for injury, it is important to anticipate the risks after transplantation inherent in living. These risks include potential exposure to others with viral or bacterial illness, to food and water sources, participation in recreational activities, resuming sexual activity, living with pets, and opportunities for travel, especially internationally. It is invaluable to orient potential SOT recipients to these risks, because often leading up to transplant they may likely experience debilitation and significant handicaps due to chronic illness. After SOT, once they overcome the preceding debilitation and surgical effects, they, despite chronic immunosuppression, can go on to live healthy, fruitful lives, which they may not have been able to fully conceive of while debilitated. Thus, in anticipation of SOT, potential transplant recipients should update their vaccinations. Potential recipients need to be made aware of food and water safety important after transplant so they may plan accordingly. In addition, potential recipients

This article originally appeared in Infectious Diseases Clinics of North America, Volume 32, Issue 3, September 2018.
Disclosure Statement: None.
Division of Infectious Diseases, Beth Israel Deaconess Medical Center, 110 Francis Street, Suite GB, Boston, MA 02215, USA
E-mail address: bblair@bidmc.harvard.edu

should be educated as to the risks of pet ownership and animal exposure, again to plan accordingly. Finally, realistic expectations should be set with regard to travel and participation in recreational activities especially within the first year after transplant, the period during which they are at increased risk of infection.[1] The American Society for Transplantation Infectious Diseases Community of Practice has previously set forth informal guidance on strategies for living safely after SOT.[2] The investigators astutely note that, unlike Centers for Disease Control and Prevention (CDC) guidelines set forth in other populations such as hematologic stem cell transplant recipients[3] and those infected with human immunodeficiency virus,[4] no such evidence-based guidance exists for the SOT population. That said, the data available for these groups and other immunocompromised populations can be extrapolated to provide guidance, understanding that this guidance may require tailoring based on an individual patient's situation.[2]

STRATEGIES TO PREVENT INFECTION
Vaccination

Posttransplant infections can have a major effect on a patient's as well as their allograft's survival; thus strategies aimed at preventing infections are likely to have significant impact.[5] One such strategy is vaccination (please see Dr Christian Donato-Santana and Nicole M. Theodoropoulos' article, "Immunization of Solid Organ Transplant Candidates & Recipients: A 2018 Update," in this issue for more details). Although inactivated vaccinations have been demonstrated safe after SOT, so too are these vaccines safe in end-stage liver disease (ESLD) and end-stage renal disease (ESRD), and antibody titer response after vaccination is higher pretransplant.[6–12] Viral infections, such as measles virus and varicella zoster virus that can be prevented by live-attenuated vaccine, can have significant morbidity and mortality after SOT.[13] Varicella disease in the immunocompromised host can lead to severe complications.[14,15] Measles outbreaks unfortunately continue to occur in the present day, and measles in an immunocompromised host can cause pneumonitis and encephalitis and has been associated with high mortality.[16]

Live-attenuated vaccines are not recommended posttransplant; thus, identifying those susceptible hosts pretransplant and vaccinating them are paramount in avoiding devastating consequences of infection in an SOT recipient. Most transplant centers have procedures in place to identify these susceptible patients via pretransplant serologies, and every effort is made to ensure vaccination occurs before transplant with intervals as prescribed by the Advisory Committee of Immunization Practices (ACIP). Two other vaccine-preventable diseases that are more common than measles require attention: influenza and Streptococcus pneumoniae. Because invasive pneumococcal disease can have substantial morbidity and mortality in SOT recipients and in those with chronic lung, heart, renal, and liver disease, the ACIP recommends vaccination with PCV13 followed by PPSV23. Furthermore, there are few contraindications to influenza vaccine in these populations, especially given the severe pulmonary and extrapulmonary complications associated with infection.[5] Live-attenuated influenza vaccine should be avoided posttransplant both in the SOT recipient and, if at all possible, in their household contacts.[17]

In general, in anticipation for SOT, vaccination should occur as soon as possible to afford protection to those with chronic heart, lung, renal, and liver disease but also because live-attenuated vaccinations should not be administered after transplant. Realistically, however, this is not always possible because in those with critical illness, there may not be time to complete vaccination series before transplant. However, transplantation should not be postponed solely for this purpose. Although the optimal timing of vaccination after transplantation is not known, most centers initiate vaccination 3 to 6 months after transplantation.[17] Despite theoretic concerns, no evidence of a link to vaccination and acute episodes of rejection has been found.[14,18,19] Thus, influenza vaccine should be administered yearly as long as at least 3 to 6 months after SOT and not given previously that season. Ideally, any encounter with a potential SOT recipient should prompt a review of vaccine status and update as indicated[5] **(Table 1)**.

Everyday Strategies for Disease Prevention

In SOT, most infections occur during the first 6 months after transplant unless there are extenuating circumstances, such as organ rejection and need for augmentation of immunosuppression. After 6 months, most infections seen in the SOT recipient are similar to those seen in the general adult population.[1] Because most pathogens are either acquired via direct contact via hands, ingestion, or inhalation, frequent hand washing and avoidance of those with respiratory or gastrointestinal illnesses are essential ways to minimize acquisition of infectious pathogens.[2] Close contacts of transplant recipients should be encouraged to receive updated vaccines as per the ACIP guidelines and their personal health care providers. There is little risk from

Table 1
Vaccine recommendations

Vaccine	Schedule	Comments
Influenza	Annually	Pretransplant & posttransplant
Hepatitis B	3 doses	Consider 40-µg dose in ESLD & ESRD
Hepatitis A	2–3 dose series depending on vaccine	Recommended in ESLD & high-risk travel
Tdap	Single dose ≤2 y after last Td	Td booster every 10 y thereafter
Pneumococcal		
Prevnar (PCV13)	Once regardless of age	If given after PSV23, then wait ≥1 y
Pneumovax (PPSV23)	≥8 wk after PCV13	If administered before age 65, then booster after 5 y
Varicella	2 dose series if nonimmune	Pretransplant only
MMR	1–2 doses depending on previous vaccination	Pretransplant only
Shingles (Varicella-Zoster)		
Zostavax	Once in adults >50 y	Pretransplant only; may be obsolete with advent of Shingrix
Shingrix	To be determined	Approved by FDA 10/20/17 & voted on by ACIP 10/27/17; official recommendations in immunocompromised hosts pending
HPV	3 doses through age 26	Catch up if not previously vaccinated as child
Meningococcal (MenACWY)	1–2 doses	Only for certain populations per ACIP guidelines & no immunogenicity studies post transplant

Data from Refs.[5,17,20,21]

family members/close contacts who receive live-attenuated vaccines to transplant recipients. The only exceptions are smallpox and oral polio vaccines, which are very rarely indicated.[17] In addition, even with rotavirus vaccine, SOT recipients could refrain from diaper changing and/or use meticulous hand washing rather than not have their close contact vaccinated.[22] Similarly, review of safe sexual practices with SOT recipients can reduce risk for acquisition of several pathogens, including hepatitis B and C, human immunodeficiency virus, herpes simplex virus, *Neisseria gonorrhoeae*, *Chlamydia trachomatis*, syphilis, and other fecally transmitted organisms. Unless the patient is in a long-term monogamous relationship, condom usage should be advised. Furthermore, SOT recipients should be counseled on avoidance of oral exposure to feces and hand hygiene after sexual intercourse.[2,3] **Table 2** lists other approaches and habits to use to avoid contact with environmental objects/individuals to decrease an SOT recipient's chance of exposure to infectious pathogens.

Food and Water Safety

According to the CDC, 48 million persons get sick; 128,000 are hospitalized, and 3000 die from food-borne infection and illness in the United States each year. The most often impacted are those with weakened immune systems,[23] which is why education and guidance should be directed at potential SOT recipients and reiterated frequently after transplantation. Waterborne infections arise from drinking contaminated drinking water or inadvertent ingestion of water during recreational activities, such as boating, enjoying water parks, or swimming.[2] Access to safe drinking water within the United States is as simple as using water from the tap delivered from and US Environmental Protection Agency–regulated public water system.[24] That said, many people in the United States who receive their water from private ground water wells are thus responsible for ensuring their water is free from contaminants.[24] The most common causes of water-associated disease outbreaks due to private water sources per the CDC as of 2010 are as follows[24]:

- Hepatitis A
- Giardia

Table 2
Avoidance strategies against environmental and opportunistic pathogens

Employ hand washing after:	Avoid:
Eating or preparing food	Close contact with persons with respiratory viruses
Changing diapers	Prolonged contact with crowded areas
Touching plants or dirt	Tobacco and marijuana smoking
Using the restroom	Visiting areas with increased risk of exposure to tuberculosis (prisons, homeless shelters, certain health care facilities)
Touching animals, particularly at zoos or fairs	
Touching items in contact with animal or human bodily fluids	Construction areas/areas of excavation
Collecting or deposing of garbage	Areas with possible exposure to fungal spores: caves, barns, bird cages/coops, soil aerosols via mulching
Going outdoors or to a public place	Self-piercing, tattooing, or needle sharing

Data from Avery RK, Michaels MG, the AST Infectious Diseases Community of Practice. Strategies for safe living after solid organ transplantation. Am J Transplant 2013;13:304–10; and Guidelines for preventing infectious complications among hematopoietic cell transplant recipients: a global perspective. Biol Blood Marrow Transplant 2009;15(10):1143–238; and *Adapted from* https://www.fda.gov/downloads/Food/FoodborneIllnessContaminants/UCM312793.pdf.

- Campylobacter
- Shigella
- *Escherichia coli*
- Cryptosporidium
- Salmonella
- *Yersinia enterocolitica*

Thus, private water sources such as these should be avoided by SOT recipients.[2] In addition, SOT recipients should avoid swimming in recreational facilities that are likely to be contaminated with human or animal waste, and if swimming, avoid swallowing such water.[2]

After transplant, many patients may experience a renewed appetite that was suppressed due to previous chronic illness such as ESLD or ESRD. Food safety is paramount to retaining an SOT recipient's health with attention paid to handling, preparing, and consuming foods.[25] Raw fish and meats should be handled on separate surfaces from other food items.[3] Separate cutting boards should be used for each food item or thoroughly washed with soapy warm water between uses for separate foods.[3] Any person preparing raw foods as an SOT recipient or for an SOT recipient should practice meticulous hand hygiene after handling raw foods.[3] Raw vegetables should be washed thoroughly before ingestion. Even fruits with skins should be washed before cutting or peeling to avoid internal contamination from the surface.[25] Canned foods should have the lids washed before opening to avoid contaminating the inner contents.[25] All cooked foods should be heated to US Department of Agriculture–recommended safe minimum internal temperatures, including reheating previously cooked foods, such as hams and deli meats.[25] These practices are simple ways to decrease risk of the many infections outlined in **Table 3**, which can have more fulminant presentations and/or be more difficult to treat and eradicate in SOT recipients. Unfortunately, many of these illnesses present similarly; thus, knowledge of potential risk behaviors can inform the SOT recipient on what to avoid, and if ill, can be highlighted to the care team as a possible source of infection/symptoms.

Pet Safety and Animal Contact

Studies have demonstrated the health benefits of animal-human bonding, especially in the immunocompromised, who may feel isolated as a result of their underlying illnesses.[28] Physicians should advise SOT recipients of the potential risks inherent in pet ownership and animal contact, although in most circumstances, such ownership/contact is not absolutely contraindicated.[3] The SOT recipient should not feed or pet stray animals. In general, pets such as lizards, snakes, turtles, baby chicks/ducklings, and exotic pets should be avoided because of risk of *Salmonella* and *Campylobacter* infections.[28–30] Specific guidance for the care of pets should include the following: feeding pets only high-quality commercial food, not raw meat or raw eggs; allowing pets to drink only from potable water sources; leashing and confining dogs to prevent coprophagy (eating feces); avoiding juvenile cats or dogs because they are more prone to enteric infections.[28] In addition, although routine veterinary care for pets is important, SOT recipients can be at risk for pet vaccines–related illness, and thus, caution must be advised. The "kennel cough" vaccine, which is a mixture of *Bordetella bronchiseptica* and parainfluenza, can pose infection risk.[28,30] The *Brucella* animal vaccine has been associated with human illness.[30] In addition to the risks potentially prevented by obtaining veterinary care, caution must be advised when providing in home pet hygiene. In general, bird cages and litter boxes should be cleaned daily by someone other than the SOT recipient. Although fish are

Table 3
Major pathogens causing food-borne illness in solid organ transplant

Food-Borne Pathogen	Commonly Associated Source	Most Common Symptoms/ Complications in SOT
Campylobacter	Contaminated water; raw meat/ poultry; unpasteurized milk	Diarrhea (often bloody), fever, nausea; can lead to bacteremia
Cryptosporidium	Contaminated (unwashed) food; contaminated drinking/ recreational water	Crampy, watery diarrhea leading to dehydration; in SOT can be prolonged
Listeria monocytogenes	Unpasteurized milk/cheeses; improperly reheated deli meats/ hot dogs; store-bought meat salads	Abdominal pain; diarrhea; fevers; chills; headache; can lead to bacteremia and meningitis
E coli	Undercooked meat; contaminated water; unpasteurized juices	Diarrhea; vomiting; certain strains can lead to hemolytic uremic syndrome
Salmonella	Undercooked meat, poultry, eggs; unpasteurized milk/juices; pet turtles	Abdominal pain; fever; diarrhea (may be bloody); can lead to bacteremia
Toxoplasmosis gondii	Raw & undercooked meats (including deer); handling cat feces	Mononucleosis-like symptoms; severe systemic disease in SOT
Vibrio vulnificus	Undercooked & raw seafood	Diarrhea, nausea, vomiting; severe sepsis in SOT
Norovirus	Contaminated food or water; close contact with infected individual	Watery diarrhea (can be prolonged in SOT), nausea, acute onset vomiting

Data from Refs.[25–27]

generally a lower-risk pet, care must be applied to cleaning of fish tanks because mycobacterial disease associated with skin and soft tissue has been linked to such activities.[28–30] Finally, after any animal contact, whether with a personal pet or at a zoo or aquarium, all individuals, but most importantly SOT recipients, should practice careful hand washing.[28–30]

Travel Advice

As per the CDC, immunocompromised travelers compose 1% to 2% of the travelers seen in US travel clinics.[31] These visit statistics are important to note because travel to destinations outside of North America and Europe are associated with increased exposure to enteric and vector-borne pathogens.[32] In a large travel clinic study in Canada from 2001, two-thirds of the travelers surveyed who were SOT recipients were foreign born[32] and historically, being foreign born increases a traveler's likelihood of staying with friends and family.[32] As such, it is unclear if foreign-born SOT recipients frequent travel clinics as several studies have indicated that those traveling to visit friends and family are more likely to contract travel-related illnesses because they are less aware of their susceptibility, less likely to seek pretravel advice, and adopt higher risk behaviors.[33–35] Because of these data, education and recommendation toward seeking pretravel advice should be targeted at all SOT recipients because improved pretravel consultation can potentially prevent devastating infections.[36] The CDC recommends that several key education points be discussed with immunocompromised travelers: developing an illness contingency plan with an identified clinic/hospital; bringing extra medications in case of travel delay; avoiding procuring medications during travel due to risk of counterfeit; use of sun protection; vigilant food and water precautions; and travel with a health kit.[31] In addition to these measures, travel to high-risk destinations should be postponed until at least a year after transplantation.[31] If a potential SOT recipient has the potential to travel to yellow fever–endemic areas after transplant, consideration should be given to vaccination before transplantation.[36] In addition, household contacts of SOT recipients can and should receive live-attenuated travel vaccinations before travel with the precautions as described above in the vaccination section.[32] As for the SOT travelers themselves, other inactivated or non–live vaccines for typhoid, hepatitis A, hepatitis B, and meningococcus should be administered as indicated.[36] In addition, malaria chemoprophylaxis should be prescribed for SOT recipient travelers to endemic areas because they are by virtue of the SOT susceptible to more serious disease.[31] Care does however need to be used when prescribing malaria chemoprophylaxis because potential drug-drug interactions with immunosuppressive medications and dose adjustment for altered renal or hepatic function need to be considered.[31] In addition, strict vector precautions should be advised because diseases like Chagas and leishmaniasis can disseminate in immunocompromised hosts.[36] Furthermore, Dengue infection accounts for about 10% of the systemic febrile illnesses experienced by travelers, suggesting that SOT recipients would be similarly affected.[37] In addition, Chikungunya and Zika viruses have emerged as important travel-associated vector-borne infections recently. Thus, information about the severity in immunocompromised travelers is still being ascertained.[36] Although such extensive travel counseling may be perceived as excessive especially by those who are foreign born, such measures may assist with preventing substantial life-altering illness by promoting travel yet in the safest way possible.

SUMMARY

Receipt of an organ transplant will most likely extend the recipient's life substantially, and, it is hoped, this extension is associated with good health. The benefits of longevity by virtue of organ transplantation need to be closely protected by education before, during, and after transplantation about potential risks and measures to mitigate such exposures. The topics addressed here ensure that an SOT recipient and their providers can plan accordingly and implement measures that will assist with maintaining such health.

REFERENCES

1. Snydman DR. Epidemiology of infections after solid-organ transplantation. Clin Infect Dis 2001;33(Suppl 1):S5–8.
2. Avery RK, Michaels MG, the AST ID COP. Strategies for safe living after solid organ transplantation. Amer J Trans 2013;13:304–10.
3. Guidelines for preventing infectious complications among hematopoietic cell transplant recipients: a global perspective. Biol Blood Marrow Transpl 2009; 15(10):1143–238.
4. Guidelines for prevention and treatment of opportunistic infections in HIV-infected adults and adolescents. AidsInfo.NIH.gov. Available at: https://aidsinfo.nih.gov/guidelines on 12/26/2017. Accessed January 1, 2018.
5. Chow J, Golan Y. Vaccination of solid-organ transplantation candidates. CID 2009;49:1550–6.

6. Keefe EB, Iwarson S, McMahon BJ, et al. Safety and immunogenicity of hepatitis A vaccine in patients with chronic liver disease. Hepatology 1998;27:881–6.

7. Magnani G, Falchetti E, Pollini G, et al. Safety and efficacy of two types of influenza vaccination in heart transplant recipients: a prospective randomized controlled study. J Heart Lung Transplant 2005;24:588–92.

8. Chalasani N, Smallwood G, Halcomb J, et al. Is vaccination against hepatitis B infection indicated in patients waiting for or after orthotopic liver transplantation? Liver Transpl Surg 1998;4:128–32.

9. Rytel MW, Dailey MP, Schiffman G, et al. Pneumococcal vaccine immunization of patients with renal impairment. Proc Soc Exp Bio Med 1986;182:468–73.

10. Linnemann CC Jr, First MR, Schiffman G. Response to pneumococcal vaccine in renal transplant and hemodialysis patients. Arch Intern Med 1981;141:1637–40.

11. Loinaz C, de Juanes JR, Gonzalez EM, et al. Hepatitis B vaccination results in 140 liver transplant recipients. Hepatogastroenterology 1997;44:235–8.

12. McCashland TM, Preheim LC, Gentry MJ. Pneumococcal vaccine response in cirrhosis and liver transplantation. J Infect Dis 2000;181:757–60.

13. Miyairi I, Funaki T, Saitoh A. Immunization practices in solid organ transplant recipients. Vaccine 2016;34:1958–64.

14. Broyer M, Tete MJ, Guest G, et al. Varicella and zoster in children after kidney transplantation: long-term results of vaccination. Pediatrics 1997;99:35–9.

15. McGregor RS, Zitelli BJ, Urbach AH, et al. Varicella in pediatric orthotopic liver transplant recipients. Pediatrics 1989;83(2):256–61.

16. Kaplan LJ, Daum RS, Smaron M, et al. Severe measles in immunocompromised patients. JAMA 1992;267(9):1237–41.

17. Danziger-Isakov L, Kumar D, the American Society of Transplantation Infectious Disease Community of Practice. Vaccination in solid organ transplantation. Am J Transplant 2013;13:311–7.

18. Kimball P, Verbeke S, Flattery M, et al. Influenza vaccination does not promote cellular or humoral activation among heart transplant recipients. Transplantation 2000;69:2449–51.

19. White-Williams C, Brown R, Kirklin J, et al. Improving clinical practice: should we give influenza vaccinations to heart transplant patients? J Heart Lung Transpl 2006;25:320–3.

20. Recommended immunization schedule for adults aged 19 years or older, United States, 2018. CDC.gov. Available at: https://www.cdc.gov/vaccines/schedules/downloads/adult/adult-combined-schedule.pdf. Accessed January 1, 2018.

21. What everyone should know about Zostavax. CDC.gov. 2018. Available at: https://www.cdc.gov/vaccines/vpd/shingles/public/zostavax/index.html. Accessed February 19, 2018.

22. Smith CK, McNeal MM, Meyer NR, et al. Rotavirus shedding in premature infants following first immunization. Vaccine 2011;29:8141–6.

23. People at risk for foodborne illness - transplant recipients. FDA.gov. 2017. Available at: https://www.fda.gov/Food/FoodborneIllnessContaminants/PeopleAtRisk/ucm312570.htm. Accessed January 1, 2018.

24. Drinking water. CDC.gov. 2017. Available at: https://www.cdc.gov/healthywater/drinking/index.htm. Accessed January 14, 2018.

25. Food safety for transplant recipients. FDA.gov. 2011. Available at: https://www.fda.gov/downloads/Food/FoodborneIllnessContaminants/UCM312793.pdf. Accessed January 14, 2018.

26. Avery RK, Lonze BE, Kraus ES, et al. Severe chronic norovirus diarrheal disease in transplant recipients: clinical features of an under- recognized syndrome. Transpl Infect Dis 2017;19:e12674.

27. Foodborne illnesses and germs. CDC.gov. 2017. Available at: https://www.cdc.gov/foodsafety/foodborne-germs.html. Accessed January 14, 2018.

28. Trevejo RT, Barr MC, Robinson RA. Important emerging bacterial zoonotic infections affecting the immunocompromised. Vet Res 2005;36:493–506.

29. Healthy pets healthy people – organ transplant recipients. CDC.gov. 2014. Available at: https://www.cdc.gov/healthypets/specific-groups/organ-transplant-patients.html. Accessed January 15, 2018.

30. Kotton CN. Zoonoses in solid-organ and hematopoietic stem cell transplant recipients. Clin Infect Dis 2007;44:857–66.

31. Traveler's health. Chapter 8 – Advising travelers with specific needs. CDC.gov. 2017. Available at: https://wwwnc.cdc.gov/travel/yellowbook/2018/advising-travelers-with-specific-needs/immunocompromised-travelers. Accessed January 20, 2018.

32. Boggild AK, Sano M, Humar A, et al. Travel patterns and risk behavior in solid organ transplant recipients. J Travel Med 2004;11:37–43.

33. Ryan ET, Wilson ME, Kain KC. Illness after international travel. N Engl J Med 2002; 347:505–16.

34. Held TK, Weike T, Mansmann, et al. Malaria prophylaxis: identifying risk groups for non-compliance. Q J Med 1994;87:17–22.

35. Behrens RH, Curtis CF. Malaria in travelers: epidemiology and prevention. BMJ 1993;49:363–81.

36. Patel RP, Liang SY, Koolwal SY, et al. Travel advice for the immunocompromised traveler: prophylaxis, vaccination, and other preventive measures. Ther Clin Risk Manag 2015;11:217–28.

37. Freedman DO, Weld LH, Kozarsky PE, et al. GeoSentinel surveillance network: spectrum of disease and relation to place of exposure among Ill returned travelers. N Engl J Med 2006;354(2):119–30.

Moving?

Make sure your subscription moves with you!

To notify us of your new address, find your **Clinics Account Number** (located on your mailing label above your name), and contact customer service at:

Email: journalscustomerservice-usa@elsevler.com

800-654-2452 (subscribers in the U.S. & Canada)
314-447-8871 (subscribers outside of the U.S. & Canada)

Fax number: 314-447-8029

Elsevier Health Sciences Division
Subscription Customer Service
3251 Riverport Lane
Maryland Heights, MO 63043

*To ensure uninterrupted delivery of your subscription, please notify us at least 4 weeks in advance of move.

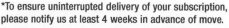

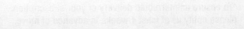

Printed and bound by CPI Group (UK) Ltd, Croydon, CR0 4YY

03/10/2024

01040477-0011